"Bless you, bless you, bless you, Judie. The world in general, and breast-cancer-concerned women in particular need this book now! *Sacred Choices* is pure delight. It will boost your immune system, enhance your mood, and in so doing help you heal the minute you begin reading it. If you or anyone in your life has breast cancer or is concerned about it, you need this book now. *Sacred Choices* is powerful medicine!"
**—Christiane Northrup,** M.D., F.A.C.O.G.
author of *Women's Bodies, Women's Wisdom,* Bantam 1998

"In 1954, when I was only two years old, my mother surrendered her life to breast cancer. I know if she had had the joy and wisdom of *Sacred Choices,* there's a very good chance that she would be with me today—sipping virgin Pina Coladas and wearing Tweety Bird slippers. I am glad to know that other mothers and daughters will have the opportunity to be blessed by this sacred and inspiring work. What a blessing!"
**—Iyanla Vanzant**
author of *Yesterday I Cried* and *In The Meantime*

"*Sacred Choices* explores new territories in style and substance while presenting a fresh perspective on illness and health. With humor, compassion and insight, Judie Chiappone celebrates life and the opportunities that confronting cancer presents. This book provides inspiration for anyone facing inevitable challenges in life."

**—David Simon, M.D.**
author of *Return to Wholeness* and Medical Director of the Chopra Center for Well Being

*Continued on next page*

"Judie Chiappone's authentic presence as a writer, healer and spiritual guide gifts us in *Sacred Choices*. We experience the exceptionally powerful and inspiring journey of her dear friend Hedy as she shares her sacred choices through cancer and beyond. This is a wonderful and compassionate guide that shows us how to live our lives each day regardless of any crisis or illness!"
—**Barbara Dossey,** RN, MS, HNC, FAAN
author of *Florence Nightingale: Mystic, Visionary, Healer* and *Holistic Nursing: A Handbook for Practice, and Rituals of Healing*

~

*The gentle art of
disarming a disease
and reclaiming
your Joy!*

# *Sacred Choices*

Also By Judie Chiappone

*The Light Touch...*
*An Easy Guide to Hands-On-Healing*

*The Light Touch Video*
(90 minutes)

*Sacred Choices for Chemotherapy*
(guided imagery tape)

The gentle art of
disarming a disease and
reclaiming your Joy!

# Sacred Choices

By

Judie Chiappone

Cover Art by Julie Dunsworth
Cover Design by Cathy Sanders
Production and Typography by Cathy Sanders


Excerpted from *The Black Butterfly,* by Richard Moss, copyright 1986. Reprinted by permission of Celestial Arts. P.O. Box 7123, Berkeley, CA 94707.


Holistic Reflections, Inc.
Judie Chiappone
P.O. Box 196129
Winter Springs, Florida 32719-6129
www.SacredChoices.com

*To Pat—*
*My Soul-Sister*

# Perspectives

- *The techniques and philosophies in* Sacred Choices *are not meant to be used as a substitute for good medical care, surgical intervention, or alternative therapy, but rather as a complement to any treatment of choice.*

- *Although all situational interactions depicted in* Sacred Choices *actually took place and portray a true story of actual experiences, the names of various people and places have been changed in order to protect the privacy of some individuals.*

- *The names of doctors and medical centers have been changed because the message in* Sacred Choices *is one of personal empowerment and spiritual connection—it is not about where one should seek treatment or which treatment should be chosen. Each individual must make their own "Sacred Choice" regarding individual circumstances.*

- *The author and the publisher specifically disclaim any and all liability arising directly or indirectly from the use or application of any information contained in this book. Any use of the information in this book is at the reader's discretion.*

- *Florida Hospital Women's Center is a shining example of an excellent community resource for providing early detection of breast cancer, and therefore, their name remains unchanged.*

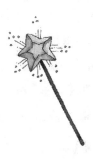

Wave that star and see
the magic in your life.
Stick end, star end...
it's your choice.

Your Sacred Choice.

# Table of Contents

*Chapter 16, continued*

# Acknowledgements

Someone once said that it takes a village to give birth to a book. Never were truer words spoken! It is such a delight to thank those who so eagerly took up residency in my village during the birthing of *Sacred Choices*.

I'm convinced that everyone should have a Pat Richey in their life. She raises the act of friendship to an absolute art form. A vigorous cheerleader, relentless visionary and "possibility thinker"—Pat has been like an "inner aerobics instructor," inspiring me to reach higher and stretch farther. She played an inspiring and powerful role in every phase of this journey. My thanks to Pat for the starring role she played in birthing *Sacred Choices,* and for enhancing my life in every way imaginable. I'm so honored to call this resplendent woman my "Forever Friend."

A huge thank you to my dear friend, Hedy Schleifer, who had the incredible insight to document the journey that followed her diagnosis of cancer. Her decision to tape our dialogues means that millions will now benefit from her amazing ability to illuminate the path of well-being during a cellular challenge and to celebrate life. My thanks to Hedy for leading by example, and lighting the way for so many others.

I am ever so grateful to Jerry and Esther Hicks who for years have showered my life with a constant flow of spiritual inspiration and clarity. Thanks, especially to Esther, for so generously sharing her ability to articulate the divine in daily life. This blend of spirit with daily life is my absolute passion, and subsequently, all I ever write about. My thanks to Jerry and Esther for the ongoing roles they humbly play in the lives of so many, and for illuminating *Sacred Choices* with the light of their love.

God placed awesome angels in my life to play key roles in this journey. One of them was Kathy Branch, a dear friend in Virginia, who somehow had the stamina, determination and talent to transcribe the hours and hours of recorded dialogue. A fringe benefit during that project stems from the fact that Kathy is one of the wittiest and funniest people on the planet. My thanks to Kathy not only for doing a superb job, but also for the side-splitting e-mail messages and fabulous words of encouragement during the months of transcribing and beyond. The fact that our friendship deepened in the process was a priceless bonus.

Another profound angel who showed up was my friend, Kay Visser. Everyone who meets Kay simply adores her. But first, you have to find her! She likes to hover in the background. Outwardly, she's extremely soft-spoken and unassuming. Inwardly, she's packed to the hilt with talent, Joy, wisdom, spiritual insight, and goodness...all of which make it seem as if you've stumbled upon a hidden treasure when you first meet her. Indeed, you have! My thanks to Kay for spending countless hours grooming and polishing *Sacred Choices,* and for being instrumental in helping me leap through every "hoop" that was somehow a requirement in the birthing process! Others who assisted Kay were Pat Richey (who enthusiastically read this book at least 133 times!), Kathy Branch, Julie Dunsworth, and Mary vonPless. These ladies were simply awesome!

Thanks to Cat Sanders, graphic artist extraordinaire, for visually gifting this book with a palpable aliveness, inside and out. It was Cat who gave birth to the beautiful "heart-vine logo" that is sprinkled throughout the text. My thanks to the "Circle of Three Publishing Company" (Jeff Tressler, Linda Seay, and Cat Sanders). Due to their generosity, I was able to use this heart-vine logo on everything related to *Sacred Choices.*

My thanks to Julie Dunsworth who so beautifully conveyed the message of "life" and "aliveness" with each stroke of her brush as she created the cover art. And, thanks to Cat Sanders for ultimately weaving Julie's art into such a beautiful cover design. God sends the very best!

A huge thank you to Dr. Christiane Northrup, Iyanla Vanzant, Barbara Dossey and Dr. David Simon for being such inspiring role models and visionaries. My thanks for recognizing the gift of personal empowerment that *Sacred Choices* offers, and for subsequently writing such powerful endorsements. They are truly my heroes!

I must thank a flock of physical angels in my village who have cheered me on during the past two-and-a-half years. My thanks to Louise Sheehey for always being there with literary blasting powder whenever I found myself stuck. Thanks to Dawn Rivera, Marjorie Brown, Pat Carter, Eileen Tatum, and Marjorie Tyler who joined me in this vision when *Sacred Choices* was merely a dream. Thanks to Gwen Meehan who continually shed tears of joy every time I took a step forward. Thanks to Dee Stone for being a fabulous role model and cheerleader in my life. Thanks to my son, Lincoln Chiappone—for reminding me to "ask" for something, even if it seems impossible. Many miracles have resulted from following his wisdom. My thanks to Karen Perce for teaching me so much about the beautiful art of giving, receiving, and celebrating life. A heartfelt thanks to the late Dierdre Brigham who was such a master at celebrating life. Her legacy continues to be an inspiration for all those seeking wholeness.

Thank you to my sisters-in-law, Jean Morse and Dee Wahlmeier, my brother, Terry Morse, and my brother-in-law, Nick Chiappone, and dear friends, Charlie Webster, George Richey, Julie Dunsworth, Caroline Owen and Donna Scharf who have all been so supportive.

Last, but not least, a rip-roaring thank you to my husband and best friend, Carl, for all he's done to enhance this journey. One of the many things I love about this man is that he always encourages me to "do my thing in life"—even if it is something he has no interest in. He roots for me to be all I can be. He enjoys my joy. And, he enhances my life with hilarious "one-liners" that absolutely incapacitate me with laughter. Carl has handled every computer-related need, and developed the fabulous new web site for *Sacred Choices*. I am so blessed to have him as my lover, friend, and partner in life. He is the reigning King of my Village!

# Introduction

Hello, My Friend,

Any idea where your magic wand is? Still have it? I'm referring to the one you received as standard issue the day you were born. We each received one. I distinctly remember how cute you looked with your tiny little fingers wrapped around your wand. What a powerful grip you had!

I know, I know... a lifetime is admittedly a long time to keep track of anything. As I remember it, you lost track of your wand the same year that you decided there was no Santa Claus. (Or was it that there was no "Tooth Fairy"? Whatever!) That was a rough year. It was the same year that the magic stopped. It was the year that a new reality set in and you began to perceive many cold, hard facts about life. Well, enough about that.

The good news is that I brought you a brand new wand, just in case you would like a little more magic in your life. You'll find it invisibly tucked right inside this book. It's yours to keep, if you'd like. Just like everything else, they've improved on magic wands since the first model came out. This one is much more accessible than your old one because you store it in your imagination. Not only is it perfect for absent-minded people (not that that's you), but it makes it wonderfully portable. The last part is critical because you'll want it with you constantly, if you want to find the fun in life. In this case, fun is synonymous with spiritual connection.

It comes with one very simple instruction:

1. Use (wave) the correct end! That would be the end with the star on it. That's where the magic is.

You automatically wave the star end in life when you say "yes!" to life—"yes" to what it is that you are wanting. However, when you say "no" to what you don't want, or push against it, you're suddenly at the stick end. You slide back and forth from "star" to "stick," depending on whatever you're giving your attention to, just like that. This doesn't mean that you can't ever say no to something you object to, it simply means don't stay there. Quit waving that stick! You've decided what you don't want, now what is it that you DO want? Put your attention there. You get more of whatever has your attention—be picky! Stick end, star end... it's your choice.

Consider that health and well-being are at the star end, and disease is at the stick end. So while you're shouting "no" to disease, or affirming that you're "going to beat cancer," the cancer then has your attention. There you are, wavin' that stick and wondering where the magic is in your life. But when you turn your attention towards health and well-being, and reach inspired decisions from that perspective, you're waving the star end, big time! While your plan of action might even be identical, there's a powerful difference in perspectives. Are you eating nutritious foods, meditating and exercising because you enjoy taking fabulous care of your body? (star end) Or, are you doing it to beat a disease? (stick end) Your body clearly knows the difference.

I look at life as one long, invisible game of "connection"— specifically, "Spiritual Connection." Whenever we tap into who we really are, we feel as if we've come "Home." And indeed we have, on an unseen level. ♪♪Honey, I'm Home! ♪♪♪ (star end) We've connected with our Authenticity. I've always had a passion for whatever would enhance my ability to sustain that connection in everyday life. I've read uplifting books, listened to inspiring tapes and attended fascinating workshops. But in most cases, there seemed to be a noticeable "gap" between the "inspiration" and the "application." There are so many distractions once you get out of bed in the morning! If you're living at the stick end of the wand, it can be awfully bumpy out there! Some jerk in the next car cuts you off on the drive to work and it's a downward spiral from then on. (Where's my wand?) Just when I hoped to "walk my talk," the gap is back! Something told me that there must be some way to sustain my spiritual connection AND hang around in regular old life simultaneously.

Well, I've found an unending supply of invisible "gap-filler." (There's plenty for you, too!) It offers perspectives about life that allow you to become a frequent winner in this game of "connection." (How nice to play a game in which everyone can win!) It's simple. It's just plain do-able. And it's right inside this book. You'll find quick and easy focusing techniques that are ideal for re-connecting with your Authentic Self and filling the "gap of the moment." The good news is, it's like working a spiritual muscle. Each time you exercise creative ways to reconnect, it gets easier the next time. (You won't need any leotards or ankle weights for this workout!)

Just out of curiosity, how would you say life is for you, right now? Does it feel like you're "doing life," or as if "life is being done to you"? Are you...

Overwhelmed with reality?
Feeling leveled by a frightening diagnosis?
Disgusted with politics?
Raging about some injustice?
Feeling tired and uninspired?
Emotionally drained by events on the evening news?

Well, it's your lucky day. <u>Sacred Choices</u> offers you a pair of celestial bifocals that will enable you to see things differently. (There's always another, "better" way to see things.) These bifocals allow you to...

take a really close look at

# the Bigger Picture!

My intention is to tease that "real you" forward into all areas of daily life, and to help you wave that star end of your wand on a regular basis. As you read this book, you'll see life illuminated through the eyes of two women, one very different from the other, yet both of whom are outrageously passionate about life and spiritual connection. You'll find inspiring examples of spirituality, joy and aliveness, not only woven into the "ordinary" moments in life, but also into some of the most challenging, as well. A parade of "wand-challenging moments" begins when one of these two women is suddenly diagnosed with breast cancer.

*"The Dance of Remembrance" (Chapter 1) is a light-hearted review of the Big Picture in life. Since we all come from varied religious and spiritual backgrounds, it is designed to embrace overall truths that bind us together beyond our differences, and show the part these same truths can play in enhancing our lives. It is a playful "spiritual massage" that lays the foundation for the incredible journey that follows.*

*It is my intention (and I hope it's yours) that you'll have your Authentic Self well in place before the end of this book (if it isn't in place already!). I have you scheduled for a fabulous family portrait to be taken at that time. This portrait will show you, front and center, grinning from ear-to-ear while standing in front of mankind. (It's obviously a wide-angle lens.) I can see it now. You look marvelous! So youthful! So spiritually connected…and did I mention fit and trim? It must be those daily spiritual workouts. On second thought, I think it's the wand and designer bifocals!*

*I trust you'll enjoy your journey as you read <u>Sacred Choices</u>.*

*In Joy,*

*Judie*

# Chapter 1

# The Dance of Remembrance

## A Spiritual Massage...
## The BIG Picture!

*Every single day, I am inspired by my epitaph. It's a "doozy"! Since brevity has often eluded me in this lifetime, I'm admittedly proud that it contains only two words. It reads:*

### "I Remembered!"

*It means that in this lifetime, I remembered-to-remember who I really was. I remembered my Spiritual Connection, or my "Authentic Self." More importantly, I remembered it right in the middle of all the chaos and drama of daily life—right in the middle of the impeachment trial of President Clinton, or while being pulled over by the highway patrol, or while having my precious dog Buttercup put to sleep...I remembered to remember! Now, admittedly, the initial brunt of offsetting events would dim my spiritual light for a bit. I worried, I judged, I blamed, I DIMMED! An aerial assessment of my shining spiritual light might have been seen as:*

*"Brilliant light—dim light—bright light...*
*Brilliant—dim—brilliant-dim—flicker-flicker...*
*Brilliant—dim—bright—BRILLIANT!"*
*(And she's baa-ack!)*

*No matter what the cause, any time my Authentic Self is short-circuited, I feel offset. (So do you.) That offset feeling signals me to "remember." My life's goal is to become faster and faster at remembering to seek higher ground; which means to think a better thought, find a better feeling, and make my way back to the real "Me." It's like celestial re-wiring. At the end of this "tour," I want to be able to boldly proclaim, "I Remembered!"*

*For me, "remembering" is as quick and easy as being aware of how I feel in any given moment. Emotions serve as my built-in guidance system. When I feel wonderful, I'm connected with my Spiritual Source. I'm connected with God. When I feel bad, for any reason, I'm disconnected. You might say that right in the midst of a life-long chat, while phoning "Home," I've suddenly hung-the-receiver-up. The telephone is dead at my end. It's a huge price to pay, and one I'm unwilling to pay if I can help it. At the moment of disconnection, I can't hear my spiritual guidance, and therefore, I'm basically out of business. The magic in life ceases. Synchronistic moments evaporate. Life becomes bumpy and a heck-of-a-lot-of-work.*

*The good news is that God NEVER hangs up at His end! But, He also won't join me in a negative thought. He can't...He knows only love. So, God patiently waits for the moment when I remember who I am, which instantly pushes the re-dial button on my phone. Presto! Once again the two of us (the Big Me) are happily re-paired and rolling along in life. (Since God takes everyone's calls simultaneously, it's undoubtedly the largest "party-line" in existence.)*

*We're putting on grand light shows as we respond to life. I playfully imagine each of us on heavenly bungee-cords of divine light. We're all bouncing around in life by virtue of this steady stream (or cord) of light from Home. But, instead of being "attached" to the bungee-cord, we ARE the cord. We are "de-light!" The very tip of this cord of light is the part we reference as "us." Our emotions operate an invisible rheostat that controls the amount of light we're emanating in each moment. The brilliance of our divine light is directly proportional to how good we feel at the moment; feeling joy and appreciation in any moment produces the brightest possible "you" and "me."*

*This light within us is synonymous with Life Force, or Energy. We open and close an invisible valve, controlling the flow of this Life Force (or Light), with our emotions. My friend, Esther Hicks, likens it to the valve in the faucet that controls the water flow at your kitchen sink. We pinch off the flow of Life Force, or close the valve, any time we are judging, worrying, criticizing, blaming, resenting, etc. But when we're loving, appreciating, celebrating, joyful, etc., our valve is wide open. So you might say that people who are angry, ornery, combative, unloving, hateful, etc., are "valvularly compromised" or they're "valvularly-challenged!" (instead of scumbag, idiot or blockhead). It works for me!*

## Affirmations for the Day:

*Nothing is more important
than that I feel good!*

*(No matter what's going on...)
I'm going to keep my valve open anyway!*

*Or, the Italian version:
"I'm-a gonna keepa my valva opena anyway!"*

*You know, it must be quite a sight from above as we each do our part in creating earthly light-shows. I think there's a good chance that it provides a gorgeous, ever-moving form of enjoyable "light-art" for the angels above. (♪♪ twinkle... twinkle...human-being ♪♪) We look up and enjoy watching cloud formations; the angels are probably looking down, enjoying our light formations! (Whatdaya think?) Even though this divine light is our very nature and synonymous with health, energy, joy, well-being, synchronicity, etc., we've come to ignore it. After all, it's invisible.*

*And we're distracted. We're busy. We're tired. Physical reality has our attention. We've got to make a living, pay bills, e-mail, shop, find meaningful relationships, restore order out of constant chaos, shop, clean the house, nurture relationships, sort the mail, fix the meals, shop, watch television, mend relationships, attend football and basketball games, look after our kids, shop...and consequently our lights are flickering.*

*Dr. Wayne Dyer once said, "You aren't what you do, or when you 'don't,' you aren't!" (Read that again!) Well, imagine with me for just a moment. Who would you be if there were no "needs" in your life that you must tend to? Imagine that there comes a day when you're done. Yep...D-o-n-e! The shopping is done...the laundry is done...no little ones need their food cut up...what's-his-name can find his own pair of matching socks...your relationships are harmonious...you're wonderfully wealthy and healthy...the house is clean...the dog is fed...there's peace on earth...everyone has a home...nothing needs repairing...you've shopped, dropped and rested (nothing needs to be returned☺)... dinner is prepared...you are sporting your perfect weight...(yep!) and your body is beautifully toned and defined. There isn't a single need in your life, or the lives of others. You're done! We're all done. Furthermore, it's a time in which credentials, titles and accomplishments are meaningless and obsolete. Who are you then? Who's looking back at you in the mirror? Who's left?*

*Most have come to think that "dim-dim...flicker-flicker" is just normal. It's just life. We think it's normal to feel crummy inside when life is just plain crummy outside. We think it's normal to resent, hate, blame, or judge, etc., especially when we know we're right about someone else's outrageous wrong! What we forget is, there's a hefty price tag tied to <u>on-going</u> negative feelings, or negative perceptions, and you pay the price with Life Force. It means we're using Life Force to keep the negativity alive (or negative perceptions alive) instead of using it to enhance our bodies as it was meant to be used. Consequently, our cellular well-being is compromised. Our cellular lights dim. Flicker... flicker...*

*So, you might say that along with the light bill most of us pay each month, on another level, we unwittingly pay a "dark bill!" Instead of being billed monthly, we're billed in the moment by our incredibly efficient "internal-billing-operations-department." I find it fascinating that the billing system for our "spiritual light" is the reverse of our electric company billing; the less spiritual light we allow in, the <u>higher</u> the price we pay. I'm personally unwilling to pay unnecessary "dark bills." I'm in a hurry. I want to continue to enjoy fabulous health, high energy, Light-heartedness, etc. In other words, I want to be who I really am, and I want to be it RIGHT NOW!*

## We're Talkin' Big Bills!

*So, you could say that along with the light bill most of us pay each month, on another level, we unwittingly pay a "dark bill!" Instead of being billed monthly, we're billed in the moment by our incredibly efficient "internal-billing-operations-department." I find it fascinating that the billing system for our "spiritual light" is the reverse of our electric company billing; the less spiritual light we allow in, the higher the price we pay.*

*Our sensitivity as to how we're feeling at any given moment means we have one opportunity after another to choose what feels better and to continually correct our course. We knew it would be an ongoing ritual in life; one that's very much like a "living prayer," the one we rehearsed before we came here. Remember? We were chomping at the celestial bit to intertwine our spiritual orientation with the fast-paced dramas in physical life. We intended for any negative feelings to merely serve as a cue that we were off-track, a cue to remember the bigger picture, a cue to think a better thought, a cue to lighten up, a cue to remember Home, a cue to live the prayer we knew so well. A cue to remember, period! It was like a little code we worked out before coming. When we feel bad, we're pinching off our connection with Home; and when we feel good, we're tapped into that divine flow.*

*Well, little-by-little, we lost our "cue sensitivity," and feeling somewhat (or a lot!) tired, frustrated, worried, bitter, anxious, hostile, judgmental, resentful, etc., came to feel normal in every-day life. After all, it's wild out there! Little-by-little, "forgetting to remember" just felt like regular ol' life. We grew desensitized and "cue-less!"*

*Looking back on my nursing career at the unending parade of symptoms and diagnoses, I would say that "cue-less-ness" was the common denominator. Just showing up for a medical exam tends to dim our lights. A diagnosis—period—tends to make us "valvularly-challenged." An ambulance ride following a coronary is a real "dimmer." But, any offsetting situation is our cue to choose thoughts or visions that steady us. (More about this balancing act, later.) While "coronary" or "myocardial infarction" is perhaps your official diagnosis, it would be more accurate to say (playfully), that you were hospitalized last week with a case of "Chronic Cue-less-ness!" Or, you might say that you were in the hospital because you had pinched off your flow of Well-being—although that would surely make some people think you're a candidate for a psychiatric consult!*

## *Soooo...*
## *Whatcha' in for?*

*While "coronary" or "myocardial infarction"
is perhaps your medical diagnosis,
it would be more accurate to say (playfully),
that you were hospitalized last week with a case of
"Chronic Cue-less-ness!" Or, you might say that you
were in the hospital because you pinched off your flow
of Well-being—although that would surely make some
people think you're a candidate for a psychiatric consult!*

*As a nurse I noticed that many times after life-and-death situations, patients were eager to reprioritize their lives and to lighten-up. The lucky/smart ones were willing to see things differently. They were willing to let go of previous judgments and criticisms that, in view of their medical scare, now seemed trivial. They were willing to forgive. They were eager to really live. Some even said that they hadn't truly begun to live until they thought they were going to die. They searched out creative ways to live more fully and add more joy to all areas of their life. They chose life and whatever supported good health, instead of putting all their energy into fighting disease. They chose approaches to their health care that "felt right for them." They chose physicians that they were in harmony with. Consciously or unconsciously, they were finally promoting the light that was, and is, their true nature. Basically, they merely reclaimed their previously diverted flow of Life Force by reclaiming their power. They re-opened their valve to well-being; they turned up their rheostat. (Pay Day!) That's called "healing." It's natural to us.*

*But back to these "valve-closers." We all have opinions and form judgments in life as we decide what we want, and don't want. Unfortunately, there's something very seductive about thinking (or knowing) we are right about someone else's wrong. It feels so correct, to feel so "right." (What could possibly be wrong with THAT!) We become not only comfortable, but downright proud of hanging on to negative opinions and perceptions, which in themselves create a log-jam in the stream of life. We notice an injustice and begin pushing against "it," instead of giving our attention to what we're wanting. We push the "save" button on our internal computer so that we can forever recall the event at a moment's notice. We vow "never to forget," thinking "remembering" will keep it from happening again, and all the suffering will not have been in vain. We flap about it and write about it. A mere reference to it unleashes a mini, on-the-spot presentation from deep within us. After all, we're right! However, we're simultaneously "valvularly-challenged" and "cue-less." And, since God won't join us in criticizing or blaming (because God knows only love), it is energetically lonely. It's the "little us" (the disconnected "us") that's out there flappin' all alone—and we've simultaneously become part of the problem, instead of the solution.*

*Here's a little "cue-test" for you. The following list of persons includes people you may know of but have never personally met, people in your own family, and perhaps people you've never heard of in your life. It doesn't matter. The important part is to just feel your way along as you read the following list:*

*President Clinton       Linda Tripp       Monica Lewinsky*

*Kenneth Star                 your father*

*your mother        O.J. Simpson        Saddam Hussein*

*Adolph Hitler             Susan Smith*

*Ellen DeGeneres          your mother-in-law (jes' checking!☺)*

*any "in-law"                 Pee-Wee Herman*

*How'd you do? Feel like spewing about outrageous behavior you associate with any of the above? It seems only normal, doesn't it? After all, you probably think (or perhaps know) that you're right! But, on an energetic level it takes a lot of Life Force to sustain blame, resentment, hate, worry, etc., by virtue of the fact that it's not your nature. You're going against your internal flow. Consider that, while your discomfort appears to be coming from whatever injustice you are focused on, it's actually produced from the withdrawal of Life Force. It's like choking off something as critical as oxygen. Hefty withdrawals are being made in your well-being account as diverted Life Force is used to support your negative perceptions instead of your well-being. Notices of insufficient funds come in by the truckloads. (You're tired, you're irritable, you have a headache, or you're actually getting sick... and, worst of all, you're "cue-less.") Sustained negativity is energetically expensive. As long as holding on to the negativity is more important than your well-being, and as long as you are oblivious to the cues, it's impossible to balance your account! This is "high finance." Is it worth it? It's your call. You may be "right," but you're also "valvularly-challenged." You have a choice. You can choose to feel better. The first step is merely to become sensitive to how you're feeling in any given moment.*

## Big Misery

*While your discomfort appears to be coming from whatever injustice you are focused on, it's actually produced from the withdrawal of Life Force. It's like choking off something as critical as oxygen.*

# A Day in the Life of a One-Minute Healer!

*While it's easy to suspect highly dramatic areas of our lives as places where we're losing Life Force, we're often oblivious to the smaller issues that are hidden in the ordinary. The sheer numbers of these tiny but "energetically-pricey" issues in the average day add up to a chronic deficit of well-being. You just never feel quite up-to-par or fully alive. Chances are, you quickly just blame it on stress and once again, have come to think that feeling this way is just "normal." It gradually sets the stage for the health problems that finally get your attention. While these issues are less dramatic and seemingly unimportant, every time you free-up pockets of diverted Life Force, it steps-up your feeling of aliveness. So, these pockets are really worth looking for.*

*Take, for example, an ordinary thing like a morning walk— something I do nearly every day of the year. What a fabulous way to begin any day. The birds are singing, bullfrogs join in on bass, the brook is babbling, fragrant flowers are blooming, the grass is greening but unfortunately—litter-ers have been littering! How disappointing. (There's my cue.) At that moment, I have a choice. I can either let litter-ers, beer cans, fast food bags, cigarette wrappers, paper cups, (symbols of thoughtlessness) etc., mess up my moment, disconnect me from "Me" and divert Life Force...OR ... I can find another way of looking at it all that feels better. I've turned this into a little game I play called "Connection!" Just as "Chop wood and carry water," is ancient advice for spiritual awakening, my contemporary version for the past 16 years has been: "Feel good, and pick up litter!"*

## Words to Walk by:

*Just as "Chop wood and carry water,"
is ancient advice for spiritual awakening, my
contemporary version for the past 16 years has been:
"Feel good, and pick up litter!"*

*So, I don my "celestial bifocals" to get a really close look at the beauty of the surroundings. As I walk, part of me is on auto-pilot, picking up litter without so much as even a judgmental whimper, while the greater part of me is programmed for any thought that feels good. I entertain myself with little private jokes about litter. My mind chuckles as it wanders and wonders about those who litter...since they throw so much out, do you suppose their cars are immaculate inside? After 16 years of "trashercise," my experience has been that Marlboro cigarettes and Budweiser beer are definitely the most popular brands. But, I muse, are these the most popular brands, or do people who are attracted to these brands tend to be more "environmentally-challenged"? I chuckle. (Perhaps I could ask for some government funding to study the* *possibilities.) I giggle. Then there are the "tidy litter-ers" who stuff all tiny condiments and napkins carefully into the paper cup, and then throw the cup! I laugh. My Reeboks are flyin' and my mouth is grinning as I entertain myself with comical thoughts—thoughts about <u>anything</u> that lightens me up! I love the honks and waves from appreciative residents that I've never met. I love seeing others who are inspired to also participate in "trashercise." I love driving out of my subdivision later that morning and witnessing the pristine beauty.*

*I wish I had a nickel for every morning walker who has said things in passing like, "Isn't that disgusting? People are so thoughtless," or "There's always some who have to spoil it for the rest of us!" etc. (Valve closed!) I smile. I translate that into their way of saying that they appreciate what I'm doing each day. None of their berating words about those who litter produce even a quiver of the needle on my animosity meter. It makes me realize how far I've come with my game of "Connection." I wish them a fabulous day, and I continue to remember to "Feel good and pick up litter!" I'll opt for more light instead...thank you! It's a beautiful day, and I'm feeling wonderful. My valve is wide open.*

*We're very creative in finding ways of interjecting negative agendas into ordinary life and dimming our spiritual lights. We focus passionately on something wonderful, and negativity sneaks in the side door. I've had this happen when telling my husband (the realist), about a new idea I'm excited about. Sometimes he'll unwittingly offer unsolicited negative data in an effort to point out any pitfalls. Poof, I'm deflated. (There's my cue!) I silently counter with the thought that he only does it because he wants the best for me. I've also learned to rely on the power of playfulness for righting myself at times like this. I take a breath, grin and quickly fire back with, "Let go of my ankle. I'm tryin' to fly here!" We laugh, he stops, and I continue to dream. My mission is always the same; one way or another, I need to get to a better-feeling spot as soon as possible.*

*But, what if he didn't stop. Or, what if it's you that's hanging on your own ankle. (Apparently you're much more limber than any of us give you credit for!) Think, hypothetically of the lovely, generous, ever-giving, cookie-baking, sweet neighbor of yours who never says a bad thing about anyone. . . a saint. . . an angel. . .and who's now diagnosed with a dreaded disease. How could this have ever happened to her? By living in an energetic "jam." It's as simple as passionately wanting something—which gets gigantic amounts of Life Force flowing—and then slamming the door shut with self-doubts or fears. The doubts can be as simple as "I'm not good enough," or "I'm not smart enough," or "I'm not enough,"—period! The fear can be as simple as "fear of failure." There you are in a simultaneous state of "stop and go," energetically stunned like a deer in headlights. Consequently, your life-sustaining, health-sustaining flow of Life Force is also "stunned." (dim-flicker-flicker) While doubt and fear are normal emotions, they were meant to serve as cues, not as lifestyles. It's not the fact that they surface that compromises us, it's the fact that we become the perfect hosts, offering them a comfortable recliner, snacks and attentiveness. With careful feeding and attentiveness, they become bigger than the dream. But, no matter what light-game we're playing, our health and well-being is always about opening to the flow of divine energy that is natural to us. The rules of the game are the same for all of us. . . even your sweet neighbor.*

*So, the only question really worth asking in any moment is, "How am I feeling?" Your emotional meter tells you in an instant whether Life Force is flowing. . .or not flowing; whether your valve is open. . .or closed; and whether your rheostat is turned up. . .or turned down. By the way, how ARE you feeling?*

## *"Wait" Just a Minute!*

*Finding a way to feel good in the moment is priceless. We have countless unenlightened stretches of "down-time" in daily life in which we wait in a powerless pause. We wait for the doctor to call or lab report to arrive, telling us if we're going to be "O.K." Most of us think that's all we can do. . .just wait. And then there's the timing. Think of how often some unsettling news arrives late on*

## *Jam Sessions!*
### *(We're often energetically jammed.)*

*It's as simple as passionately wanting something—which gets gigantic amounts of Life Force flowing—and then slamming the door shut with self-doubts or fears. The doubt can be as simple as "I'm not good enough," or "I'm not smart enough," or "I'm not enough,"—period! The fear can be as simple as "fear of failure." There you are in a simultaneous state of "stop and go," energetically stunned like a deer in headlights. Consequently, your life-sustaining, health-sustaining flow of Life Force is also "stunned."*

*a Friday afternoon, and we spend the weekend doing the "worried limbo." We review every "What if?" we can think of, leaving nothing unturned. (dim, dim, flicker!) The same goes for any stretch of time in which we have to "wait it out." Perhaps you get the final news, and it isn't good. For example, your lab work results show that you are clearly moving in the wrong direction, and your health is at risk. So now you're trying to live with that, and "that" is the last thing to focus on when you want to live! (You might want to read that again!)*

*Well, there's "waiting"...and there's "Waiting." In the first case, you are disconnected from your spiritual source (silently begging, hoping and bargaining while focusing on fears and concerns). But in the second case, you are spiritually paired and in the flow. The "enlightened you" knows the power and benefit of feeling good about something...anything! You know that on a cellular level, good thoughts bathe you in well-being. You also know that it's the perfect tonic for every condition and situation. You know that this tonic instantly enhances every single cell in your body.[1] You also know that it is only in this state that you can hear spiritual guidance.*

*The "enlightened you" has a long list of options that immediately change the game. You know how to deliberately crank up your flow of Life Force. It's as easy as finding a thought that feels better. As far as yesterday's lab results, that was then, but this is your "precious now!" So, in THIS "now" you rummage through your Spiritual First Aid Kit and choose something that feels better. It contains a long list of wonderful touchstones (it's a big kit):*

- *Laugh uproariously about something—anything (Television sit-coms are wonderful.)*

- *Take a fabulous power-nap. (Sleep reconnects you.)*

- *Meditate.*

- *Begin writing a list of things you appreciate.*

- *Begin sifting through your memories for things and events that open your "valve" big-time! Dig treasures up from the past, "re-love" them in your "now."*

- *Sniff-out a judgment (or negative perception) you didn't know you had and let go of it... unleashing Life Force.☺ (It's like finding a buried treasure!)*

- *Turn on a movie that makes your heart sing.*

- *Play a game of positive "what if's"—"What if I sail right through this and I'm given a clean bill of health?"*

- *Have a massage.*

- *Have an energy-balancing treatment and celebrate the magnificence of your body.*

*In other words, "lighten-up!"*
*Given what the medical community has come to know about the mind/body connection, and that our bodies are continually responding to our thoughts and emotions, this decision to move to a better-feeling spot is a powerful one. It means that in THIS moment, on a microscopic level, you're already enhancing your body's well-being. In other words, the data is already looking more favorable, even if current tests are unable to measure it.*

*You're already moving in the right direction. That can be quite a comforting thought in the middle of the night.² Having ongoing sensitivity to the way we feel, is the way that we were meant to live our lives. In living by the motto "Nothing is more important than that I feel good," and using techniques to re-connect on-the-spot, you've just become the "One-Minute Healer!"*

*Moving away from "cue-less-ness" and towards connection, requires practice. I love practicing "valvular aerobics" during television newscasts. They provide such a handy slice-of-life and are usually easier to process than the relationship issues of family and friends that hit closer to home. Ever notice how disconnecting the 5 o'clock news can be? (And the 11 o'clock news...the 6 a.m. news...all newscasts for that matter.) It offers such a rich blend of connection with disconnection. I find it downright fun. What better place to practice staying centered while seeing wild snippets of life. I slip on my celestial bifocals to take a really close look. I revel in all bits of heartwarming news. But for the sensationalized, unpleasant footage, I practice looking right through it all and on to a better way to see the situation. There is <u>always</u> a better way to see anything. Admittedly, there's often an "I dare You," paired with my request for guidance to inspire me with a better vision. ("I dare You to unravel THIS one!") God, Christ, Holy Spirit, Buddha, angels—(whomever YOU turn to) all love a perceptual dare, and I have never been disappointed in the response. It's about seeing another perspective within a perception...a story within a story. It's also about remembering to ask! The rules of this game of mine are simple. When I am able to look r-e-a-l close, and emerge feeling good...I win! And after years of practice, I'm thrilled to say that I win a lot.*

*Now, it's not a game of calling "black"..."white." It doesn't mean that I look at horrendous pain someone is enduring and think it's wonderful. I have merely learned to see <u>what else</u> is going on—other than the pain, suffering and "wrongs" in life. For example, in the Oklahoma bombing, I quickly began noticing the enormous parade of people reaching out to help others—people who were perhaps giving of themselves in a way that was beyond* *anything they had ever extended to others prior to that event. "Authentic Selves" were surfacing everywhere, as people were being enormously kind and helpful to others. And, I noticed people being willing to receive help and comfort—people who had possibly never allowed themselves to "receive" before. Most of us have flunked previous courses in "Receiving 101" or never stopped to register for the course in the first place. It's times like these that give us a crash course in honoring ourselves. In seeing the bigger story and finding things that feel better, I am able to be of help. You can either be of help, or join the chain of pain. It's always your call.*

*No matter what offsetting news surfaces, I have programmed myself to stay at it until I feel better. (Even if it takes days.) I have a make-believe computer software program inside me (Perceptual Windows '00), well backed-up on a huge floppy disc. If I experience a momentary internal crash, I can promptly re-boot my program.*

*But I don't stop after looking beyond "the obvious" in the story. I take it a step further. For any offsetting news, I busy myself sending e-mail without a computer. I send "energetic gifts" in the form of uplifting visions and prayers of encouragement. I bathe these people (people I'll probably never meet), in peace and well-being. I send visions of them regaining their connection, their balance, and most of all, their spiritual aliveness. It is my knowing, as it rolls off my heart and mind, it arrives instantly as a gift for them. If they are unable or unwilling to let it in at that moment, my gift remains with them until they are willing to feel better...until they are ready to open their e-mail. It surrounds them in the form of "grace" and will be there to steady and uplift them when they are willing to let go of the pain and move forward.*

*I watch the news almost every single day. These days, I can watch an entire newscast and maintain my connection. I must warn those of you at home not to try this "alone"—without your "Celestial Bifocals." Unless you're paired with your spiritual connection, the stimulus is sure to be hazardous to your well-*

*being. . . the perfect time to utilize the "off" switch on your remote. But if you want to try it, be sure to put your request in ahead of time to see it differently. Then lean back and enjoy this spiritually-enhanced version (vision) of the news. There's a bigger story there!*

# *Will the Real Me, Please Rise!*

*Over the years, I've become aware of how many "me's" there have been. "The girls," I lovingly call them, one for each phase of my life, one for each passionate focus. It has given my husband the sensation of having had several wives all in the same marriage. Luckily, he says that he likes the current one best of all, so far, knowing that there will likely be more to come. Looking back, I can see now that the driving force was my passion for "Authenticity" (sounds like a lovely name for a girl). No matter what had my attention, I wanted to feel that connection with the real me.*

*I'm a recovering Catholic (actually 20 years Protestant, 20 years Catholic, and the past 17 years, a Free Spirit). I spent years living from a perspective of being a "good person" so that "I'll get to Heaven." However, patience has never been a virtue of mine. That old "waiting for Heaven" business seemed awfully long—especially since I plan to live a very long life. But, then I came to realize that we don't have to wait. We can let Heaven flow through us right here and right now when our "valves are open," our "rheostats are turned up," or we've "lightened up." It's a wonderful thought, isn't it? It just means that we simultaneously open to the divine energy from Home when we find ways to feel good.*

*I love the fact that Heaven is so portable. I have it with me while standing in line at the dry cleaners or while at the beauty shop coloring my hair. (You'd think after 35 years of regular bleaching that my hair would just give up and willingly grow out blonde!) But, where was I? Oh yes, the flow of Heaven. So each day, I just do my best to "be it!" or to "be the flow." My day is like*

*one long chat with God. The sky and earth form my cathedral.
You, and everyone else make up my congregation. (Sometimes it's
a rowdy service.) Frogs and birds frequently serve as the choir for
the day. The service never lets out.*

*Among other things, I'm a Registered Nurse and Licensed
Massage Therapist, healer, and author. I've coined the term
"Nursage" in my work; intertwining professions as I enhance the
body, mind and spirit of others. I love giving them the deepest
massage possible—that of massaging their very soul. Ummmmm.*

*My passion lies in:*

- *Illuminating the true nature of others...*

  - *Celebrating the Authenticity in myself and others...*

    - *Continually seeking Joy
      (synonymous with spiritual connection)...*

      - *Never doing anything unless it's fun
        (definition of fun = fully-connected spiritually)...*

        - *Delighting in the ability to enhance someone in
          France while I'm vacationing in Fargo (or, was
          I vacationing in France while enhancing someone
          in Fargo? Whatever!)...*

          - *E-mailing without a computer (sending
            invisible energetic gifts)...*

            - *And celebrating the One-ness of us all
              (particularly delightful as I contemplate
              that "I am one with Tom Selleck.").*

*You might call it a daily "Dance of Remembrance." I dance
anywhere and everywhere—while bagging potatoes in the
produce department of the grocery store, or while standing in line
at the ATM. It's a world of expanded awareness overlaid on the
mundane, making it life in the fun-lane.*

*I lovingly claim the title "The Queen of Fluff," adoring the
invisible/spiritual element in life...that data-free, fat-free,
hard-to-measure, but nevertheless profound fluff. I'm currently*

*celebrating 36 years of marriage to Carl whom I have dubbed, "The King of Data and Logic." This is the man who, while I was in labor, was compelled to chart my contractions on a graph. And later, as our son began formula feedings, another graph would appear on the inside of the cabinet door to quickly determine the ratio of powder to liquid. I fluff him up and he grounds me. It's a rich blend of realities. Well, at times it might be described as a temporary collision of realities—nonetheless, we repeatedly surface as best friends and lovers.*

*Years ago, Maurice Chevalier sang a song in the Broadway musical* Gigi *that was titled, "I Remember, Yes I Remember."[3] Carl and I laughingly call it "our song." Perhaps you know the one...*

*"We met at 9..."*
*"We met at 8..."*
*"I was on time..."*
*"No, you were late..."*
*"Ah yes!...I remember it well!"*

*...two ongoing realities within the same love-nest.*

*Carl's passion is softball and I'm the self-proclaimed head cheerleader. Since I'm often the only person sitting in the bleachers, it's not hard to pretend that I am the head cheerleader. His team is called "Cheers" and the games are delightful. I love it when Carl instantly snags a hard-hit ball while playing third base. That "theuppp" sound is so satisfying. The delight is quadrupled as he quickly throws to another base for a second out, and I now have one puffed-up, adrenaline-pumped Italian. With continued errorless playing, the ride home in the car is guaranteed to be a mobile play-by-play review as he delights in re-loving the game plays.*

*But then there are those "other games" which are filled with major disappointments, and the ride home in the car is the equivalent of a "self-flogging mobile" as Carl beats himself up about errors he made and opportunities he missed. Yet, I find myself, "Miss Fluff," riding along side of him but with most of the game plays already mushed together in my mind. Those bumpy-sporty-moments are now "unretrievable" from my data bank. I personally enjoyed the game. We each witnessed the very same event, but Carl's miserable and I secretly had a good time. I say "secretly" because this would definitely not be the moment to tell Carl about how much I enjoyed myself. When someone's having a bad day, there's nothing more annoying than being around someone who is flapping about major happiness and joy. While I won't join him in his distress, I also won't flaunt my well-being. Timing is everything.*

*Win or lose, my enjoyment of the game has to do with the long list of things that I find to appreciate. I like noticing the personal effort of individual players—that impossible catch, caught! Or noticing how close they come to catching one. I love the banter between the catcher and the batter. I delight in seeing the "little boy" peeking through the persona of each player (all of them 50 years or older) as they take their turn at bat. I love the softball humor, like–"Bury me with my bat and glove…just in case!" At the end of each game, I never cease to find it fascinating that the throng of players spread all over the field, magically form two opposing lines out of total chaos, exchanging "hi-fives" with each player of the other team. "Good game" they chant to each other. (Indeed!) I love sitting in beautiful, sunny Florida in December—sporting my t-shirt, shorts and Reeboks. Florida is my kind of climate. Life is good. These things (and more) sustain me even as Carl vents his frustrations and his "if only I could'uvs." Upon arriving home, he's soon busy on the computer recording game statistics and contemplating his next game plan. I smile. Fluff and Logic, quite a pair!*

*A sign on a telephone pole once read:*

### *LOST DOG*
*Has 3 legs*
*Blind in left eye*
*Missing right ear*
*Tail broken        Recently castrated*
*** Answers to the name of "Lucky"*

*Perception—yours, mine, theirs, and Lucky's…isn't it great? We're always free to choose the way we personally perceive life. This fact alone, accounts for the myriad of truths. I've come to know that there can be more than one truth. Like the three blind men describing an elephant. One has a hold on the tail, one has the belly, and one is grasping an ivory tusk. Their descriptions about what an elephant looks like vary tremendously, yet each is correct.*

*Personal perceptions and philosophies in life may vary but the goal is usually the same. Most of us want to run the bases in life swiftly—while reaping joy and delight along the way—sporting a spiritual aliveness during the run, and grinning from ear to ear from all the exhilaration as we return to "Home Base" to score that final run. (Can you remember if it's possible to do "hi-fives" in Heaven? Or does your palm pass right on through theirs? I'll have to check on that.) One of the fascinating things about senior softball is that the rules require two "home plates" in order to avoid collisions. The catcher runs to one plate while the player runs to another plate a few feet away. Different paths, same home. This is precisely how I see all our different philosophical versions of "The Truth" in life.*

# A Perceptual Massage at Camp Diversity

*If you'll think back, there's a good chance you'll remember a time when you and I really spent a lot of time together. It was quite a long time ago, back before we were born. We were totally clear about who we were and that we were direct extensions of God. We knew that we were the very tip of a steady stream of God's light. It was a wonderful time in which:*

- *There were no support groups or support hose.*
  - *Everyone had a matching pair of socks…even the men.*
    - *There were no wrist watches, or neighborhood watches,*
      - *No fat-free diets, Viagra or fears…*

- *No crutches, canes, pollution or zoos,*
  - *No 12-step programs, contact lenses or war,*
    - *No waiting lines, state lines, boundary lines, parking lines or frown lines.*
      - *We all flew "Etheric Airlines" and our baggage was never lost!*

*Our alphabet was a little different then.  It began with the letter "B," BACDEFG...It was a reflection of our knowing that "nothing we <u>do</u> is ever as important as how we <u>Be</u>!" So we gave our friend "B" first billing.*

# Human Beings... or Human Doings?

"Nothing we <u>do</u>
is ever as important
as how we <u>Be</u>!"

*We spoke a little differently then. You might say we spoke the language of "Well-being." It was one of empowerment. It celebrated our True Selves—our Authentic Selves—wholeness, balance, steadiness, Spiritual Connected-ness, abundant Life Force, joy, clarity, flexibility, freedom, etc. (You remember!) We were filled with delicious descriptions of what we loved and wanted more of. Our vocabulary oozed with many of the same words we use today:*

| | | | |
|---|---|---|---|
| love / loving | appreciating | | willing / willingness |
| liking | confident | knowing | admiring |
| radiating | joining | sparkling | resplendent |
| accepting | connecting | energizing | |
| imagining | thrilling | exhilarating | celebrate |
| en-joy-ing | wonder | wonderful | |
| ecstasy | co-create | healthy | |

*passion*   *profound*   *playful*   *delight*
*invigorated*   *expanded*   *growing*
*enthusiasm*   *stunning*   *remarkable*
*adventurous*   *uplifted*

*There was a steady, unending supply of Joy. It's no wonder because Joy is the infallible sign of the presence of God!*

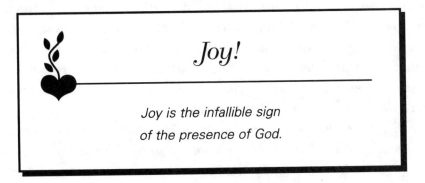

## Joy!

Joy is the infallible sign
of the presence of God.

*We would playfully refer to each other with royal-sounding titles such as "Your Joy-ness!" Everyone knew the value of never passing up a chance to have fun.*

## The Jewish Talmud[4]

"When you reach the gates of Heaven,
you will be questioned on all permissible pleasures
that you have not partaken of."

*So, what does all this have to do with you and me and our lives today? Well, as I recall, we made it very clear before we ever set foot here on earth that our top priority would be to sustain that same spiritual connection as we rolled around in all the diversity here. It seemed simple enough. We'd just do what we had always done before—we would notice contrast for a brief moment, and then immediately turn our full attention towards what we wanted more of—because we get more of what we give our attention to. Furthermore, we said, "Since God is Joy...and each of us is a direct extension of God, it will be easy to know when we are connected and when we're not. We will merely feel our way along. When we feel joy (or goodness, or appreciation, etc.) we'll know we're connected. Our sensitivity as to how we are feeling in any given moment will guide us. Fear, doubt, worry, resentment, blame, etc., will all be cues to 'turn the other cheek,' meaning find another way to look at the situation. Negative emotions will be a cue to find another way that feels better, a way that re-pairs us with our spiritual connection." We called it "celestial pivoting." (It's the current dance of remembrance.)*

*But then came the surprise. Who knew we'd get so caught up in "reality" and that we'd be so captivated by the contrast. A mere sixty seconds of a painful verbal exchange with a "valvularly-challenged individual" can stimulate hours, and even days, of regurgitating the event. We focus and re-focus on the outrageousness of it all. Bad news (e.g. a frightening diagnosis), belittling words, a perceived failure, etc., can dis-empower us for weeks, months, or even years—whatever length of time we choose to keep the spotlight on it.*

*The reason this is such an important point is that many of us spend every waking hour reacting to "negative stuff" in our day. "How can I ignore it?" you say. "It's everywhere!" (Surprise, surprise!) It's like a dog that's chasing its tail and missing the juicy porterhouse steak a few feet away. ♪♪♪ "Here boy! ♪♪♪ Over here!" ♪♪♪*

*In relationships, we often find ourselves thinking that "if only they were more like us," or "if only they'd see things my way," or "if only they'd behave differently," then things would be better. All the while our gaze is fixed firmly on what we're not liking. But, here's a question for you. Have you ever considered the possibility that we chose this earthly experience specifically because all those variables existed? Or that we chose all this contrast because it's so stimulating for our soul? And that we purposely came here to be exposed to different tastes, smells, sights, sounds, touches, climates, geographical locations, relationships, truths, opinions, cultures, behaviors, careers, body shapes, colors, clothing, etc.? We didn't say prior to coming here, "Get it all perfect," or "Make it all the same," or "Create peace on earth," or "Get everyone to think like us," or "Get everyone to love everyone,"—and then we'll come. It was all the diversity that actually called to us. We said eagerly, "The more the better!" "Let's go!" Suddenly, we found ourselves in a group that had formed on the "leading edge"— spiritual volunteers for a rich, spiritually expanding, potentially entertaining, temporary human experience.*

*The difference between life back Home and life here is that in the non-physical we were masters at giving our full attention to only <u>what we were wanting</u>. As my friend Esther Hicks puts it, we looked at life much like you'd look at a cookie counter that's packed with all kinds of cookies to choose from. We'd eagerly search for our favorite ones (chocolate chip) and then trot off with a bunch of them in absolute delight (Did I mention that we could eat and eat and never get fat?) with never a reference from our lips or hearts about the peanut butter cookies that we didn't care for. We didn't begin worrying that the peanut butter cookies would multiply or overtake the cookie counter. We didn't spend time contemplating ways in which we could confiscate the remaining peanut butter cookie dough, or the recipe so that no more could be made. We didn't try to keep the peanut butter cookies out of the cookie counter. We didn't spend time pushing against their existence. We merely noticed that they weren't for us and filled our cookie bag with our mouth-watering favorites. Since we automatically get more of whatever we are giving our attention to—we knew that our "thrill" over chocolate chip cookies automatically placed an order with the celestial baker for more of the same. (Conversely, trying to exclude peanut butter cookies would give them our full attention, and we would find them showing up everywhere. Oooh, there's another one over there!) Once again, it's not about painting black—white, or painting chocolate-brown spots on peanut butter cookies so they'll pass for chocolate chip.*

*It's not about denial. And, it's not that you shouldn't use your talents to make a positive difference in the world. It has to do with whether you are pushing against the problem, or embracing the inspired vision of how it could be. What's your attention on? It's a matter of focus.*

*Well, here we are, playing out our lives at "Camp Diversity," softly mumbling, "If only I could have it <u>my</u> way." We're ever-pressed to "face reality!"—especially when it comes to an unexpected dance with a life-threatening disease. We notice good cookies and bad cookies. In actuality, as we bump up against anything unwanted, the most appropriate thing would be to shout, "Cookies! Just more cookies!" and "Let's see, I'll have the macadamia, chocolate-chip, frosted ones, please. Yummmm!"*

## *Reality!*

*Never, never face reality...*
*unless you really, really like what you're seeing.*
*In that case, give it your full*
*and undivided attention!*

# Chapter 2

# Cookies!

## (From Life's Cookie Counter)

*It's such a pleasure to introduce you to a dear friend of mine. A woman who is truly gifted with a clear knowing of "Home" and who has an ongoing affinity for all that is sacred. At a time when so many are seeking profound self-discovery "up there" and "out there," she is finding the profound "right here." At a time when many admittedly think that negativity in day-to-day life is just normal and that the game plan for life is to tolerate it the best way you can ("This is as good as it gets!"), this woman sees negativity as a cue. It's a "wake-up-cue" to immediately seek a better-feeling spot, think another thought, look at it another way, or make another choice. (Sound familiar?) It's her cue (and hopefully yours, too) to immediately head for what feels better... without looking back...and without dragging toilet paper (negativity) on her foot as she runs towards the light.*

*Anyone experiencing even brief moments of "her" knows that something wonderful has transpired. She provides a touchstone that simply feels delightful. Her steadfast tenacity for feeling good, results in a life that many refer to as "charmed."*

*She laughs,*

*she dances,*

*she prays,*

*she admires,*

*she travels,*

*she loves,*

*she is loved,*

*she praises others,*

*she sings,*

*she raves,*

*she questions rules,*

*she breaks rules,*

*she entices,*

*she inspires,*

*she clarifies,*

*and...*

*she heals.*

*The question is, does life just come to her charmed? Or does she <u>charm</u> life! I think you'll soon see that it's the latter.*

*As the "Magnificent Hedy" (pronounced "Hay-dee") puts it: "God (the Kosher Choreographer) gives us time and space. It's up to us to fill it with meaning and Joy."*

---

## *A "Hedy-ism!"*

"God (the Kosher Choreographer)
gives us time and space.

It's up to us to fill it
with meaning and Joy."

---

*This woman breathes so much Joy and meaning into her life that it has surely spilled over into future lifetimes. She's a master of Joy and of being fully present in the ever moving "eternal now."*

*Although we first met in 1988, it feels as if I've always known her. Ours is one of those friendships in which we pick right up where we left off no matter what amount of time has passed between visits. You might say we operate on "eternal de-light time."*

*I love watching her pull into my driveway in her bright red Lexus. She slowly emerges from her car in such a purposeful exit. She's usually adorned from head to toe in lots of fabric; often a middle-eastern look with a large scarf draped across her bosoms and fashionably thrown over her shoulders. She loves dressing up and wearing large, unique jewelry. It's normal to see at least six rings on her fingers. (Being a person who wears absolutely no jewelry most of the time and who's favorite outfit is a t-shirt, shorts and Reeboks, I find this all fascinating.)*

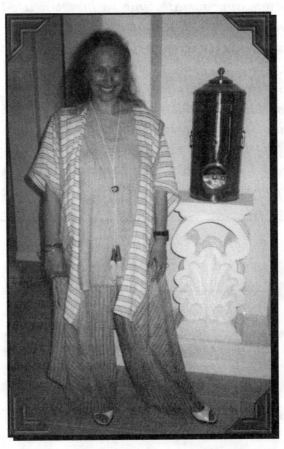

Hedy

*She moves with passion and a style that is all "Hedy," sporting a long, intentional stride that has the flavor of royalty. Massive curly gray hair ("big hair" as she calls it) floating softly as she makes her way towards my front door. Her body is tilted back slightly, pointing her bosoms to the heavens. Simultaneous Oh-ing, Ahh-ing, Oy!-ing and laugh-ing begins the moment we spot one another. We eagerly exchange an exuberant, full-body hug. Two excited women so fully-present that it turns a regular visit into an event! Our time together is always magical.*

*It's safe to say that most people who know Hedy tend to babble in admiration just as I have. Her radiance spills onto those around her wherever she goes. All of the above makes for quite a "ségue-challenged" moment in this story—for there just never seems to be an appropriate time to insert a life-threatening diagnosis into one's life. But, to put it simply, there came a day when an uninvited visitor slipped quietly into Hedy's experience. This visitor would not only dramatically affect Hedy, but all of us who knew her as well.*

*It was in March of 1997 when Louise, Hedy's best friend, was to bear the unbelievable news. She had no more than settled into the flannel sheets on my massage table, when she confessed to having a very heavy heart. She had news that our mutually treasured friend, Hedy, had just been diagnosed with breast*

## Cookies!

*We're ever-pressed to "face reality!"—
especially when it comes to an unexpected dance
with a life-threatening disease. In actuality, as we bump
up against contrast the most appropriate thing
would be to shout, "Cookies! Just more cookies!"
and "Let's see, I'll have the macadamia,
chocolate-chip, frosted ones, please. Yummmm!"*

cancer. Absolutely stunned, I stood listening to the details of what "they" (the physicians) had said, and how Hedy was handling it.

For a few moments, breathless waves of disbelief, injustice and compassion cycled through my heart. Other feelings flew through me too quickly to identify. It was a flood of everything I've ever known about cancer and an instant recollection of every person I ever knew who had been diagnosed with it. Awful feelings (there's my cue!) poised for "retrieval" at times like this. I found them neatly filed in my internal data bank, exactly where I had last left them. I could hear and feel them simultaneously. It was admittedly a breath-taking chunk of emotional inventory.

When I consciously resumed breathing again, a nice deep breath served to soften this un-welcomed scenario. The next breath allowed me to reclaim my spiritual connection. I love that "place"...that "me"...that steady, loving, calm me. There's such magic in that spot. Fear disappears. Fear or love...I can focus on one or the other, but it's impossible to do both at the same time. That means that my decision to intentionally find that loving space or to seek higher emotional ground is a power-filled one. I had shifted, I was reconnected, I was ba-ack after a brief but wild trip.

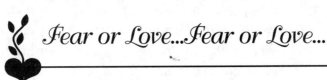

### Fear or Love...Fear or Love...

Fear or love...
I can focus on one or the other, but it's
impossible to do both at the same time.
It means that my decision to find that loving space or
to seek higher emotional ground is a power-filled one.
I had shifted, I was reconnected, I was ba-ack!

I knew that I really wanted to be of help. I began energetically flavoring Louise's massage with a silent message that "All is well," as I worked. Deepak Chopra describes human beings on an energy level as moving around in an invisible "air soup." We can *and are reaching others who are miles away with our thoughts and our intentions. I loved knowing that from miles away Hedy was also receiving this same gift, this steadying message that "All is well!" Word of Hedy's diagnosis spread rapidly throughout our community to friends all across the continent and Israel. A push of the "send" button on e-mail and presto, hundreds knew of "the news." Friends everywhere quickly mobilized to assist her in whatever way possible. A lot of them were engulfed in anguish over what appeared to be a "sneak attack" in the night on their dear friend. They saw Hedy as the victim of a dreaded disease. It seemed to subconsciously mirror their own perceptions of just how vulnerable we all are. This was just too close to home for many of them.*

*Friends said over and over, "Hedy, I'm here for you. Call me if there's just anything you need or if there's anything I can do." Although they sincerely meant it, they energetically had their arms wrapped around the painful news and their fears. They felt helpless. They mentally paired Hedy with the diagnosis, thinking, "Poor Hedy has cancer." While sincerely wanting to be of help, they unwittingly joined the chain of pain and weighed-in on the side of the fear. Even though these are very normal responses, the greatest gift we can give anyone who is teetering after any emotional blow is the gift of empowerment. That can only be accomplished when what you're feeling inside matches your words outside. You've got to get into a good feeling spot within, in order to truly offer the touchstone that they are intuitively seeking.*

*I was eager to send her a gift. It was in the form of a letter, just the kind of letter that I'd want to receive if the situation were reversed. I wanted the gift to be in writing so that she would have the opportunity to feel it's message over and over again as she read and re-read the words. I designed it to empower, uplift, and steady Hedy. It was filled with a simple reminder of how to reign-in your Authentic Self at a time when life appears to tug us powerfully towards everything we're not. The gift of Empowerment... it was the greatest gift I could offer.*

# *"Heart Prints" in the Mail*

*It definitely stood out amidst her huge stack of mail that day. The envelope was addressed to The "Magnificent" Hedy Schleifer. Miniature opalescent doves (confettios) were tucked inside and poised for stimulating unexpected delight. I had tucked the letter inside a greeting card that had a picture of a toddler wearing a bright colorful bandana on her head that was tied in a huge knot. She was sitting on a little chair—totally engrossed in examining her own bellybutton! A snippet of life at it's best.*

*My letter was as follows:*

March 7, 1997

My Dear Magnificent Hedy,

This is your Magnificent Friend Judie, sending a huge, invisible gift, designed to cheer-on the fully empowered Hedy! I am a self-appointed member of your support team, invisibly surrounding your heart (and Yumi's) with my heart. From miles away, I am launching the energy of profound Well-being and Joy—aimed straight for the two of you...don't duck!

Here's my "four cents" on the subject of fabulous health. In your mind's eye, picture a gorgeous, golden, magic wand...the wand of life. No assembly is required and no batteries are needed. However, it does come with a set of very clear instructions.

1. Use the correct end! (It's the one with the star on it.) Many people are waving the stick end in life and wondering where the magic is!

2. The star end is what you are wanting more of...the stick end is what you are not wanting.

3. You get more of whatever you give your full attention to...just like that!

Devastating news can often make the best of us "wand-challenged" for a bit. The trick is to limit your attention to brief periods when you're focusing on what you're NOT wanting...then pour all your attention into what you DO want. The gift in a distasteful diagnosis is that it helps you quickly and clearly discern what it is you are wanting...perfect health! It provides a powerful springboard for a fabulous launch.

I'm aware that you are "well-launched" so-to-speak and busy moving in the direction of a pro-active plan. All that in "wand-eze" means that you are at the magical end! Hoo ha! However, if you bounce back and forth, engaging both ends of the wand, it neutralizes your efforts. Here are some examples of each end of the wand.

- "I really, really love the feeling of a healthy, vibrant body." (star end)

- "I was diagnosed with cancer." (star end)

- "I have cancer." (stick end)

- "I'm experiencing a temporary cellular challenge." (star end)

- "I love taking excellent care of my body." (star end)

- "Why me?" (stick end)

- "I'm going to beat this disease." (stick end)

In attempting to "beat the disease" you automatically give "it" your full attention which potentially keeps you from moving forward. Instead of trying to "beat the disease" it's more productive to celebrate life in creative new ways. For example, you exercise just because you love taking extraordinary good care of yourself and you're worth it… not because you have to beat a disease. There's a big difference in how your body responds between the two scenarios.

You come with a built-in "wand sensor." When you feel good (joyful, happy, silly, blissful, peaceful, etc.) you are at the star end, and when you feel bad (worried, angry, frustrated, guilty, resentful, etc.) you're at the stick end. The idea is to play any game that makes you feel good, and know that, on a cellular level, your cells are instantly responding with changes that promote good health.

I love lying in bed at night and imagining that each cell in my body has a very bright light and that I'm shimmering from head to toe. Even my eyelashes sparkle. I enjoy taking an inventory of all my internal organs and systems and seeing everything brightly lit. My heart sparkles as it beats, my blood is shimmering as it flows, my lungs sparkle as I inhale and exhale, etc. Imagine the tremendous flow of Life Force that's actually being celebrated within every cell during that vision!

I use the memory of my dog Buttercup to instantly re-connect me any time I feel offset by situations or events. Just having her invisibly with me, massaging the little webs between her toes (the Labrador Retriever in her), stroking the soft part of her face, etc. Bingo! I'm at the star end of the wand. Music, art, nature, and pictures I've torn from magazines also fill my personal "Life-Force First Aid Kit." Nothing is ever more important than that I feel good. Only then am I allowing Life

Force to enhance my body. Only then am I fully connecting with my Spiritual Support Team. (God won't join us in blaming, worrying, fearing. Instead, He waits patiently until we are willing to give our attention to loving thoughts.) The only way we can truly be of any real help to others is to take care of our inner selves first. It's like on airplanes when the emergency instructions tell us to put our own oxygen mask on before assisting those around us.

I send you and Yumi fabulous insight, strength, and the knowledge that this whole scenario contains a huge gift, wrapped in breast tissue. Along with whatever medical or surgical intervention you are "inspired" to choose, find every creative way to choose and celebrate wellness and wholeness. Dance the medical dance only long enough to gather beneficial data and then twirl off towards what you are wanting. You never benefit by being at war or fighting against what you are not wanting. This is the dance of remembrance...the dance that awakens you more fully to the truth of your being. It has a profound rhythm to it. Listen for the beat of life. Watch for every possible creative way to put your attention fully on joy, health, and life.

And, when friends are anxious to help and ask if there's just anything they can do, say, "Yes! Please take one or two minutes here and there each day to imagine me enjoying my perfect health and well-being. Associate the mere mention of my name with words like 'healthy, vibrant, amazing, steady, fabulously-alive, strong, and sparkling'. And hold thoughts of me paired with tremendous cellular harmony, cellular giggles, sparkling light in every cell, and Life Force flowing abundantly throughout my body—big time! That is the greatest thing you could do for me!" (Unless they also *do windows!) Count on me for doing exactly that (but not the windows!).*

*There is enormous love here for you! Call me anytime you want me to rattle off more of the same.*

*In Joy,*

*Judie*

To my delight, this letter of empowerment provided a spring-board into major togetherness for the two of us in the months to come. Hedy was inspired with the idea of recording her story as it unfolded, and wanted to tell it to me. As a result, this was the beginning of hours and hours that the two of us would spend together taping delicious dialogues. It would also give birth to one of the most beautiful stories of Spirit being blended with the most challenging of times. Even when faced with a diagnosis of cancer, Hedy is a master at remembering to yell, "Cookies!" Her epitaph many years from now could easily read, "I Remembered, Too!"

Hedy's story is about making "conscious choices" and about "yes-ing" her way through life.

It's about:

- choosing what you are <u>wanting</u>,
  - choosing what you <u>will</u> have,
    - choosing life,
      - choosing to "selectively sift" through disconnecting medical data, e-mail and get well notes,
        - choosing health,
          - choosing your "dream team,"
            - choosing the inspired course of action,
              - choosing the perfect (chemo) therapy cocktail,

- *choosing to speak the language of Well-being,*
  - *choosing to see right through the lab coat and into the "human being,"*
    - *choosing to celebrate regularly along the way,*
      - *choosing to notice synchronicity,*
        - *choosing to give thanks often,*
          - *choosing to look for rules to break and protocol to stretch,*
            - *and eventually, choosing to find cancer boring!*

*This story is not about what type of therapy anyone with a similar diagnosis should have. Each person must look for whatever he or she is inspired to say "yes" to. But it is about a woman who dares to remember who she is in the midst of breath-taking news and throughout the journey that followed. A woman who dares to coax others into remembering who they really are—whether they are dear friends who are fumbling for comforting words, or doctors and nurses offering their professional care. It's a simple story about "Life by Touchstone," our earliest form of Braille.[1] It's the story of a woman who feels her way along with abundant simplicity; a devout Jewish woman who dares to remind everyone that "All is Well."*

# Talking to the Spatula

*Less than a moment after pressing "play" on my answering machine, I heard the unmistakable exuberant voice; that rich Belgiun, Jewish-Mama accent, enunciating to perfection—words punctuated with a distinctive Hedy-rhythm.*

*She said, "Ju-die Chia-ppo-ne, my magnificent friend. This is the magnificent Hedy! I cannot begin to explain what your letter has meant. I mean, this wonderful letter arrived at a time when I was 'doing this without naming it.' I was intuitively feeling my way along, finding ways to feel good about this journey. I had decided I was just going to make this a splendid, splendid adventure. I knew that I was already moving along, but your letter arrived and just propelled me forward. I want to get together with you very soon for a visit. Yumi (Hedy's husband of 34 years, pronounced U-mee) and I have had miracle after miracle in our lives. I want to tell you about this incredible experience and put it on tape as it unfolds because this is quite a journey!"*

*To my absolute delight, within a week the familiar bright red Lexus was once again pulling into my driveway. The "news" seemed to have heightened our thrill (if that were possible) of being together again. Arms locked firmly around each other's shoulders; me—never missing a chance to playfully mimic her stride—we "strode as one" into my kitchen.*

*It's a "happy kitchen" with hot pink counter tops, white cabinets, white tile, a high ceiling, large windows, and hot pink striped cushions on white barstools. It has a playful candy store feeling to it. We settled at the kitchen table that looks out into an array of flowers, trees, hedges, birds, squirrels, and armadillos. Nature at its best.*

*Preparing for this record-setting visit was not only delightful but also technically challenging. Since I had only one lapel-microphone, I realized we'd somehow have to share it as we recorded our conversation. I began searching for something that I could attach it to so that we could quietly pass it back and forth. I found the perfect tool in my kitchen drawer—a white, rubber-tipped spatula. I clipped the microphone securely to the rubber tip. It quickly seemed both perfect and hilarious at the same time. Two excited women pouring their hearts out for hours and hours to a spatula! It somehow added to the fun and served as a continual reminder not to take ourselves or life (or death!) too seriously. As the weeks progressed, we became eager to share this dialogue with others. The spatula became a metaphor for "spreading" the gift of empowerment that emerged from "a gift wrapped in breast tissue." A gift that would come to remind us all of our first (but forgotten) language, the language of Well-being.*

# Chapter 3

# Rallying 'Round the Boob!

Once past the initial shock of the diagnosis, Hedy's playfulness gradually re-surfaced like a welcomed old friend. Awestruck by the seemingly instantaneous parade of family and friends who surfaced to support her, a Hedy-ism was born. She referred to all the fanfare as, "Rallying 'round the Boob!" One by one, friends came to form an invisible scaffolding under, around and through her. Soon she was dubbing each one of them a Charter Member of "The Boob Brigade!" These same people later would give a whole new meaning to the term "support." Months later, a thousand women who were gathered for the annual Woman's Interfaith Prayerfest would sit spellbound by her story as she appeared before them with her husband, Yumi. She gazed into his eyes and said softly, "During these past months (increasing in volume), **you held my hand in a way I didn't know a hand could be held.**" (He, of course, was the first Charter Member of "The Boob Brigade.")

**Note:** Before you read the dialogue that follows, it's important that you have some awareness of the expressive ride that Hedy can take you on when you hear her speak in person. Although you'd immediately detect a slight accent, she speaks fluent German, French, Spanish, Hebrew, Yiddish and English, making it almost impossible to pinpoint her ethnic origin. One minute she might project her voice into the heavens, and the next minute sink *to a faint whisper. She* loves *to* whisper! *She weaves these highs and lows in with a charming "grammatical free-lancing" that slides all over the place. It's quite a wonderful ride as she carries you from experience to experience, and perception to perception.*

*To simplify the format, I've used a change in fonts to indicate which one of us is speaking:*

> *When I am speaking, it's written in Italics.*
>
> When Hedy is speaking, it's written without Italics.
>
> *Cues, such as [laughter] and [playfully], have been sprinkled throughout the dialogue to further invite you into the intimacy of each moment.*

*Ready now? With hands firmly joined together across the kitchen table, a "grinning duo" is filled with eagerness to birth this story!*

*Well, here we are speaking to a white spatula. [laughing] What a vision! Oooh well, first of all, let's just close our eyes and bless this time we're going to spend together. Uhmmmm. [softly]: As we settle into this wonderful moment, I want to call in our invisible angels—the girls: Flo(w), Clarity, and In-spi-ra-tion! We ask that this offering be choreographed from on high as we speak from our hearts and minds. Amen.*

**Yes. Amen!** That was just wonderful. Well, I'm so eager to tell you this story because at every juncture, God was holding us in Her palm!

*I was going to add that! [laughing]*

Although, you know, Yumi says God is a couple! He's convinced **God is a couple!**

*[sinking to a near whisper]:* Well, this all began when we got this diagnosis which, at that time, was certainly bad news. You know, I've really seen the distinction, better than ever, between news, bad or good, and then the event that you are embracing. When it's good news you get all excited and everything, and then you need to center and embrace the event. And when it's bad news, you get all flustered and overwhelmed and worried and scared, and then you have to center **and embrace the event!** So it's actually...

*[in exuberant unison]: Ex-act-ly the same! [laughing]*

But you know, we don't think of it this way, and others don't either, because, for them, "it's news," you see. For me, this news has quickly become an old story—and I'm so much further along with it in my life as a result. But when we got the news, we sat in our living room and allowed ourselves to just "see who showed up."

## The Poignant Pause

*When we got "the news,"
we sat in our living room and allowed
ourselves to just see who showed up.*

And who showed up was a friend of ours, Ted, who is a doctor and a wonderful friend. So we called him, and he said, "You know, it so happens that the person who is now the dean of the medical school here is THE nation's authority on breast cancer, and he has written a book on breast cancer." This was just very reassuring because THE nation's authority just showed up, and it was clear that our friend could easily create an

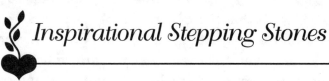

appointment for us. That was really very inspiring. It was just the reassurance that everything we needed was going to be put in front of us.

*No holds barred.*

No holds barred. If we needed THE nation's authority, that person would just be given to us! After that, Ted sort of showed up a number of times on the telephone. We eagerly told him that he was "rallying around the boob" and that he was part of the "Boob Brigade," along with many others that have become part of this adventure. So we've had "charter members" of the Boob Brigade and others "grand-fathered in" to the Boob Brigade. *[laughing]* And I mean, people have just played with this thing. Ever since then, Ted has been leaving messages like, "This is your charter member of the Boob Brigade calling!"

## The Mammogram...
## of Mammograms!

Well, it will be three weeks ago tomorrow that I went to have my mammogram. I just went the way I went anywhere. Ta dum, ta da, ta dum, ta da, ta da—you know, making a connection with everybody as I passed through. This Florida Hospital Women's Center that our dear Alice MacMahon created, is such a fabulous place.

*I've been there. Yes, as a matter of fact, I've been there and it was a wonderful, or should I say, smashing experience!*

Ah, yes, smashing! Anyway, it's such a lovely place and the women on the staff there are just marvelous! They are such advocates of screening, breast exams, mammograms and all of that...

*...and teaching.*

Teaching, teaching all the time. The nurse palpated my breast, which I love. I love lying there and having that done...so gentle and loving and nurturing. I mean, these women are phenomenal. The nurse examining me didn't feel the lump because it's so small. I was told that one in 50 women, over the age of 50, are getting breast cancer—and I thought casually, "Yeah, okay." So then I went into the mammogram thing and you know they squash it so **flat!** I'm always laughing with this thing, this pancake, you know they make it into a pancake!

*I've often thought that, given the breast tenderness that some women have who have fibrocystic conditions, the pain produced when they flatten the breast could cause them to pass out! Surely, for a couple moments they could be suspended there by one breast! I'd think that even as quickly as the technician could press the release button, they'd still never look the same again after that! [double laughter]*

You know, in gratefulness, I have written a letter to many who have helped as part of my Boob Brigade. One of the letters that I will be writing soon is going to the radiologist who interpreted my mammogram. Unbeknownst to me, this radiologist had met me two years ago when I had a benign cyst. Somehow, he remembered me and also that Alice MacMahon was a good friend of mine. When he saw the lesion, he immediately called Alice at the Women's Center.

*Uhmmm!*

He also called the surgeon to find out how I was after I had learned of the news.
*Incredible.*

This anonymous man, in a small dark room with mammograms...!

*Just like I was saying, it's so wonderful to know, that right in the middle of high-tech chaos, there are pockets of this "connected-ness" alive and well where people are "fully present" and functioning from their heart!*

Pockets! Absolutely... so I have written to that man to let him know that I know, because you know, otherwise **he'll never know that I know!** He'd just continue to do his work with the mammograms in that darkroom, unaware that I found out how much he cared and how much his thoughtfulness meant to me. So, unbeknownst to me, these phone calls were going on about "How do we tell Hedy?"

And so ultimately my gynecologist received the message and is the one who called me on Monday. She called my secretary and said, "Take Hedy out of her session. I have news for her." My secretary was smart enough to say, "Oh no. If you have news for her, I am not taking her out of her session. Let her finish and then I will tell her." (This was brilliant.) However, for the half-hour that my secretary had between the phone call and giving

## Fear Food.

*"Rather than feeding each other's delight in this woman's next 'growth opportunity,' they feed each other's fear."*

me the message, she had time to get utterly terrified. So by the time she came to me, she said, *[breathlessly and in a state of panic]:* "Hedy, your gynecologist...you have to call her right away...she has an urgent message for you." (The thing that also happens when these phone calls go on, is that people feed each other's fear. Rather than feeding each other's delight in this woman's next "growth opportunity," they feed each other's fear.)

But, I thought (speaking slowly and softly), this – is – the time – to – slow – down. I am not joining this hysteria. I am about to get some bad news. I need to receive it in my center. I-will-**not**-rush-into-this. I will **not**. You know, how often do I get bad news? I'd better be there! Woody Allen once said, "Everybody dies, I just want to be there when it happens."[1] I thought, I want to be there when this news happens. I'm not going to get numbed with urgency. So, I took my time in returning her call. When I called, my gynecologist said, "You'd better come right away."

And I said, "You know what, I am not coming right away. *[slowly and lightly]:* I – will – come – when – I – am – ready to – come!"

Then I thought, what do I really need to do? I knew I needed to do something to get centered because I could feel my skin... you know, all the fear responses were there...fast breathing, my skin got flushed, my heart was pounding. Then, a perfect touchstone came to mind. Oddly enough, something magical had happened in my office just the week before. There is a young man that I have been assisting, who has had a diagnosis of severe ADD (Attention Deficit Disorder). When he was nine years old he started coming to me for psychotherapy. He is now 21 years old and I have accompanied him through this period of his life. The week before, he came in with his mother and brought this enormous "boom box," twice the size of your stereo. He proceeded to clear my room. He cleared all the chairs and said, "Sit here on the floor." I had no idea what was going to happen. I sat on the floor as he asked. He had a big bag with him. He put on his martial arts clothing, his black belt, and out of the bag came a black belt which he held draped through his open hands, as though offering a gift. And he had a piece of paper with him containing notes written in Japanese. (He had studied Japanese and now speaks it fluently.) He had his mother sit in a chair, and began playing Japanese drum music in the boom box. I'm sitting there thinking, "What is happening here?" Well, he holds this black belt and he says, "Dear Hedy...(in Japanese, and his mother is translating, and the drums are playing) this is my first black belt. I am giving it to you, because **you are a master healer,** and the black belt master healer of the eighth degree." (This is all in Japanese—the drums are going. His mother is translating.)

He says, "This is not an award or a recognition, this is a fact, and this black belt just describes this fact. You have followed me. You have believed in me. At times when my life really was tough, you held that position of the "best" in me. You have done this for so many people, and therefore, today, I pass on this belt. And before I pass it on, I will put it against the sweat of my forehead that holds all of my spirit and strength, and give it to you with all of my blessings." (Meanwhile the music is playing, the mother is translating, and I am sobbing. I cannot believe this is happening.) And he passes this black belt to me.

I began to thank him and he said, "You know, there is really nothing for you to thank me for, this is just how it is."

So I thought, this is what I am going to do. To center myself, I will tell this story to my staff. They had been curious about the black belt that had been on my desk all week. I kept telling them, "Oh, it's a long story," and I never took the time. Now was the perfect time. And this was the perfect story for each of us.

I called in my staff, and they were like, nervous, you know. "What's going on?" they asked. And I said, I want to tell you a story. And I took all the time in the world to tell the story of the black belt. It bore such a priceless gift for everyone. I really needed the reminder that I am a healer, because I suddenly needed to heal me and everybody around me. More than ever before, I needed to remember the truth about myself. And this young man had, just the week before...

*Provided the perfect touchstone...*

The perfect touchstone.

The story was told and was precisely what each of us needed. Feeling much more centered, I went next door to Yumi's office. Yumi was out of the office for the afternoon, but I went to see Pat, his office manager. And, I said, "Pat, I just want to tell you something. I am slowly going to get some bad news *[laughing]* and I just want to hold your hand." And so I held her hand, and when I felt ready, I got into my car.

To my delight, as I drove on to Maitland Avenue, God smiled and sent a train! You know, one of those e—nor—mous ones *[in unison]* where it's one wagon after another. And, I just sat there going, "Okay...I got it. Just stay centered, and go slow."

*And steady.*

And steady. When I finally arrived at the doctor's office, God had been busy again! There was this little boy, probably three years old, on the other side of the glass door. He wouldn't let me in! There is this glass door, and he's looking at me, laughing, and I'm trying to push the door, and he won't let me in. He's laughing and I'm laughing, and I'm thinking again, look..."Another opportunity to slow down, center, and even laugh a bit." Who

---

*Slowing Down for the "Show-Down"!*
*The Kosher Choreographer Again!*

*"And as I drove on to Maitland Avenue,
God smiled and sent a train! Then when I arrived
and tried to open the door of the office building,
God sent a little boy to pretend
he would not let me in!
Okay...I got it.
Just stay centered and go slow."*

better than this little boy to make it into a little game. I mean, he was just precious, laughing and saying, "No, you're not coming in here." And I laughed and said, "Yes, I am coming in there!" "No, you're not coming in here." And we're playing this game. It was such a welcomed interlude.

*Nothing like a purely-connected little soul to clear the way, and to remind you who you really are. What a great connection!*

Exactly. Completely. Like that! *[snapping fingers]* And children, of course, have that complete and perfect total innocence, you know. So, I went in and I suddenly see my gynecologist. She looked terrified. And I said to her, "Let me hold your hands for a moment. I know you have bad news for me, but you must take a deep breath, because you have to be centered like I am, when you tell it to me. I do not really want to hear your fear. I just want the news."

*Perfect.*

She was very grateful, and she took a deep breath. We went to her office and we held hands, like you and I did before we began this recording. She took another deep breath, and then she said, "You know, your mammogram shows a lesion that looks like it is probably malignant. I want you to go to a surgeon right away." And she says, "My very favorite surgeon of all times is unfortunately on maternity leave and not available." In retrospect, that was a big blessing—that she was on maternity leave—because had I gone to her, I would have stuck with her because she has such a good reputation. And, I wouldn't have searched for what I searched for. I would have just said, "Let her take care of me, instead of WHO is going to take care of me."

*You would have given your power away.*

Yes. I would have gone to her and all her associates there, and been thrilled to be in connection with this group. But no, she had to be on maternity leave. The Kosher Choreographer was at it again!

Another favorite referral of my gynecologist was actually a woman who had come to see me as a client, so I knew her very well. We are good friends. And I said, "Fine. I can't think of a better scenario than to go from friend to friend, on this day."

So she called her and was told that I could go right over. Yumi arrived just at that time and so we went together. And again, we paused together to center ourselves. We forgot just one little detail. We forgot to pick up my mammogram films—just a little detail, like the diagnosis, I mean, who cares? *[laughing]*

*Perhaps the Kosher Choreographer was at it again?*

Absolutely. So Yumi went to get the films. It provided the perfect time to just sit there and take some really deep breaths. Time to ready myself inside for the next step.

*Uhmmm, leave it to you to see this block of time for the gift actually provided...we can deliberately choose to use it in ways that promote our wholeness and well-being. Or, we can use it to spiral downward and self-destruct! But we always have choice in the matter. Along with the goal of wanting to feel better, the perfect question to ask ourselves as quickly as possible is, "What's another way I can look at this?"*

 *The Perfect Question!*

*Along with the goal of wanting to feel better, the perfect question to ask ourselves (as quickly as possible) is, "What's another way I can look at this?"*

"What's another way I can look at this?" Exactly. And that is precisely what I did. I thought, you know, at this point, I don't know anything yet. There is a suspicion that it is malignant, but I really don't know yet. We'll figure this one out when we get the results. That felt better.

*A little breathing room—some welcomed space!*

Welcomed space for sure. Yumi was back shortly with the mammograms. My friend showed us the difference between a lesion that is cancerous, and one that is a benign cyst. That's very interesting, because a lesion that is cancerous does not allow the blood in. It has a firm circle around it, and it has a bit of a shadow because the blood doesn't come into it. A cyst has like a halo around it because the blood comes in and out, and there is light. So she says, you know, this little one, (pointing to the film) really does look like what we suspect it is—a malignant lump. And this one, which we have been watching, is really a cyst. And, she showed me the difference. Yumi and I looked at each other and we said, "Um, okay, so it looks like it is malignant."

To my delight, she was able to do the biopsy that same day, and I was on the table in no time. I got a local anesthetic. She pinched me a few times and it still wasn't numb. It takes me a long time to get numb because I am so conscious. My whole body is so conscious! *[laughing]* I am always checking everything out...and my boobs are conscious too! They wouldn't go to sleep! They're saying, "What do you think? Shall we go to sleep, or not?" And so it took a long time. They do the biopsy with something that's like a gun. They stick a needle right into the lesion, so that they know where to shoot this gun. The gun has a little serrated saw and they go "pp-ttuu" and that saw goes in and...

*How did that go again? [teasing]*

"Pp-ttuu!" I'm telling you, it sounds like a real gun! I really didn't feel much of anything. She went in seven times with that gun.

"Pp-ttuu, pp-ttuu!" And each time she pulled out some tissue. For most of the time, I didn't look, but at one point I thought, "I am really interested in seeing it." Well, it turned out that it made me nauseous. Sometimes it is not a good idea to look! You know, I am so curious about everything that goes on in my life. But anyway, she took the thing out, and I actually felt fine afterwards. I mean, I felt really fine.

*[whispering]:* So Yumi and I decided we're going out to dinner and we're gonna play tonight because we are getting some news that is gonna mean a major re-direction. We might as well just take time with each other in a very, very loving place. So we went to a place downtown that we love, called Le Provence. I don't know if you've ever been there, but listen to this story. As we go in, we hear *Enya* playing, which is Celtic music—beautiful—and there is nobody else in the restaurant.

They show us to a table and the waiter says, "Are there just the two of you?"

And I said slowly, "Well, it's the two of us and a host of angels!"

He says, "Really? Why?"

I said, "Well, we really need angels swarming around us tonight."

He says, "Oh, well, that will be arranged."

Every waiter came to swarm around us and they said, "We're the angels." Over and over they just came and served us. There was nobody else there, so they just continually focused on us. I began crying.

I said, "Yumi, do you see what's happening?" I mean, it was like they knew.

Then the music changed and it was Frank Sinatra. But, I was not in the mood for Frank Sinatra, so I said to one of them, "Would you do something for me? Could you see if you could find that other tape and play it over and over again? Because it's just perfect."

"But, of course," he said. In minutes, *Enya* was delighting us again. We stayed alone and were served by these swarming angels 'til dessert. And that dessert! It was incredible. Other people started coming in, and Frank Sinatra came back on and we were done. It was time to go.

I said to Yumi, "This is the way this whole thing is..."

*Orchestrated for you.*

Orchestrated! By the millimeter! We went home and we called a few people. But, we really called from a place of fear, confusion, concern, worry, and aahh! overwhelm. That was really the place we were in that night even though we had noticed the angels and everything. We were just like, "What are we going to do with this one?"

Tuesday morning was again filled with more magic. Now listen to this. I was supposed to go to New York on Tuesday for a wedding, a very special wedding that I didn't want to miss.

I said to my physician, "Can I go to New York tomorrow?"

And she said, "Well, if you feel fine, of course."

So, we called the airline to confirm the time our plane leaves, but we can't get an answer because there is a recording that says, "Don't forget to bring your identification. Don't forget to bring your identification." And it's, like... stuck!

And I say to Yumi, "Did you find out when we are leaving?" And he says, "No, because there is this message, 'Don't forget to bring your identification.'"

Anyway, he finally got it. Five o'clock in the morning, we get up, we get ready. My friend Louise comes with Frank at 5:30 a.m. just to say goodbye and bless us, and I say to Yumi, "Yumi, I'm not going to take this bag. All I have in there that I might need is my driver's license—I'm not going to drive a car. And you have your identification."

So, we get to the airport and...

*They—want—your—identification! [laughing]*

They said it thousands of times! I wasn't meant to go to New York. It was so phenomenal. It was an angelic hand guiding me. You know, "Leave this bag and your identification behind, because you're not going to New York!"

*[continuing in a whisper]:* We came back home, and we needed to be home. We needed to be together. We needed to take it slow. We needed to center ourselves. We didn't need to be on a plane to New York, in the cold of New York, talking to seven thousand people at a wedding—we didn't need to be there. But the beauty of that divine orchestration…that hand, guiding us! *[reflecting and shaking her head]:* You'd think that we would have gotten it! "Take your identification." They said it a thousand times. But no, I wasn't meant to go. So well choreographed!

*And the real beauty is that you recognized the scenario as being guided to perfection by an unseen hand, rather than the perception of "now our travel plans are a mess!" You saw it for what it was.*

Right away.

*It's so tempting to get wrapped up in trying to "make things happen." Trying to hammer it through, despite the odds, despite the rules, despite the one thousand reminders to bring your identification! Instead, you promptly spotted angels at work in your life.*

Right away. I said, "Yumi, look at this! It doesn't matter how much the world tells you to 'take a vacation'…if the angels don't want you to go, you're not going to go. Period!" We needed to be home, and we just relaxed and went to sleep. We were actually quite tired, quite tired. We slept and then we woke up and then we had a light meal and then we slept a little more.

Early in the following week, we finally got "The News." The diagnosis was indeed cancer. You know, we were prepared to receive that diagnosis, if necessary. What we weren't prepared for, and what came as a shock, was a spiel that was paired with the delivery of the diagnosis. A spiel that, for a time, knocked me off my center.

So there we were with my doctor. She is lovely, and she loves me. So it's like, there is absolutely no intention on her part other than to be the best physician she can be, as she takes care of me.

*It's the best she knows to do.*

She truly is the best, and she gave me the best of the best, but it was the following:

"What we have found is that this tumor is malignant. It is cancerous. And, fortunately, you have options. And your options are: to have a lumpectomy, which is the removal of the lump and the tissue around it and the removal of all of your axillary nodes; or you can have a mastectomy, which is the removal of your breast."

She said that if I chose a mastectomy, there is something wonderful they now do with reconstruction. I mean, it actually looks like your own breast. They actually take the fat of your belly and move it up. It's called a tram-flap. They make it into a breast, and then they fashion a very real-looking nipple.

And, she said, "When looking down you will not be able to tell that one is the reconstructed breast. AND...you get a tummy

## The Spiel

*Early in the following week,
we finally got "The News."
The diagnosis was indeed cancer.
You know, we were prepared to receive that
diagnosis, if necessary. What we weren't
prepared for, and what came as a shock,
was a spiel that was paired with the delivery
of the diagnosis. A spiel that, for a time,
knocked me off my center.*

tuck in the bargain. AND, according to the research that I know of, the survival rate of those people with a mastectomy is somewhat higher than the survival rate of those with a lumpectomy."

Visions, options, and a new diagnosis swirling in my head. I played it back again and again in my head…it was like… *[talking in a fast staccato]:* Boom! On the table. Lumpectomy, mastectomy, you can get a little tummy tuck. Let me make an appointment for you with a plastic surgeon so you can find out everything about a reconstructed breast! *[Hedy's hand slaps the table as a final "boom!"]*

*[softly and slowly]:* I am sitting there. I haven't even digested the fact that actually there's a lump in there that's gone a little wild, you know, it's started a little vagabond dance…I'm not even digesting this, I'm not even having the language for it…I'm already being told that I have two options, and one is actually more attractive; it's the one where I can have a flat stomach and I can have a new boob, and I will survive better with that one. The thing makes no sense. The whole thing makes no sense to me. I'm sitting there going, "This makes no sense…It's probably not even true." And I was right. It's not true. But I knew it. I knew it wasn't true. For that, I am so proud of myself. I sat there and Yumi sat there and the two of us looked at each other, and it was like, "Nah, we need a lot of study."

*Timing is everything, isn't it! I know she must have felt good being able to offer a list of options that she thought were the best. It's such an individual thing. Other patients might have been pleased to move right into the "options list" at that same moment. Options that would "fix" them up good as new.*

Absolutely. Anyway, she said, "Look, I am leaving town for a week, but when I come back I'm already scheduling you for another biopsy of the cyst and then we will just do whatever you have decided."

Okay. She had to be taken out of town, *[laughing]* which is so amazing. Because, given our friendship, and given the fact that she's an outstanding surgeon, there would have been a bit of pressure there to...

*Comply.*

Comply at some level, after all, she knows what she is talking about and she's good. And she has my best interests at heart. And she is my friend. But, she has to leave! ☺

*The Kosher Choreographer at it again, making sure you moved on to other possibilities that you would resonate to whole-heartedly. I can picture Her smiling from above at the outrageous response that this scenario produced deep inside you! Your whole body was humming with the "knowing" that this package wasn't for you. Thank goodness you listened on the inside!*

   *If you look at all the choices available in healing today, all of them work for some people, some of the time, but not all of them work for all people, all of the time. Some heal by having surgery, some by foregoing surgery, some do a combination of things, some do nothing. There's a lengthy list of what has been given the credit for healing others: chemotherapy, radiation, herbs, medicines, acupuncture, supplements, prayer, forgiveness, love, visualization, hands-on-healing, massage, meditation, etc. Some use a combination of several alternative choices to successfully heal. But, no matter what combination is chosen, the most important ingredient in the healing process is the person themselves and their sensitivity to how they are feeling in any moment. They are the healer! It's that old "open-valve" thing again, that we've talked about. They've got to feel their way along, as they have conversations with physicians, read medical data, talk to others, etc. They've got to be quick to notice anything that "closes their valve," just as you did. Then, they must recognize it as a powerful cue to seek higher ground, and utilize any creative means they can think of, to feel their way back to "wonderful." It's from that perspective that the best decisions are made, guidance can be heard, and healing has already begun. And, it's from that per-*

*spective that they are able to choose the treatment they personally resonate to that is best for them.*

You're absolutely right...and we did just that!

When we left her office, we looked at each other. Where do we want to go now? The answer was: we want to be on top of Orlando, the very highest place we could think of. There is a beautiful restaurant in downtown Orlando that is located on the 28th floor. It seemed like the perfect spot. The only problem was that it was closed. We said to the man at the door, "Well, we know you are not open...we just want to sit here for a little while."

"Well, you really can't," he said.

"Really? We can't? *[softly appealing]:* We're not going to, you know, do any harm here. We've received some news we need to process, and it would mean so much to sit here. We just want to be on top of Orlando."

"Oh. Well, okay then."

You know, people just...

---

## 🌿 *Surprise...You Are the Healer!*

*If you look at all the choices available in healing today, all of them work for some people, some of the time, but not all of them work for all people, all of the time. No matter what combination is chosen, the most important ingredient in the healing process is the person themselves and their sensitivity to how they are feeling in any moment. They are the healer! It's that old "open-valve" thing again.*

---

*Throw open the doors for you!*

Throw open the doors. So we sat there and we just said, "We're on top of the world here. We don't really know what we're going to do with this, but we need to be on top of the world. We will be on top of the world, but we don't feel on top of the world yet, so let's just stay here until we are!"

*Until your "valves" are wide open!*

Precisely. And we really did. We watched Orlando from the top, and took in the view and the sunset. And we made a list of people to call that night. We thought, "Tonight we're still in shock, and who are the people we should call?" So we made a list of the ones we thought would be the right ones to give us a hand. You know, there are people you don't call in the middle of your trauma because they'll just add to it...and there are people you can depend on for help.

One person I decided to call was a young doctor in New York who is gay, and I performed his commitment ceremony to his partner. It was an unbelievable ceremony. We have been friends for a long time. I am basically the one who helped him come out of the closet and helped his parents to really embrace him. And I performed his brother's wedding ceremony, so it's like I am part of his family.

And so I called him, and I said, "Michael, this is the diagnosis, etc." And he said, "Tomorrow morning you call my friend Allen in Atlanta. He is my mentor. In the meantime, I will call Allen and tell him, 'The Queen is calling you' and 'You take good care of the Queen.'" And of course, Allen is like this major doctor, BUT I'm the Queen! *[laughing]* I went to sleep knowing that would be the first call of the day.

We called Allen the first thing next morning, and there was again the gift—an angel. Allen gets on the phone, and I mean, he's this doctor with lots of experience and sounds very authoritative, almost sergeant-like. "So, what's the diagnosis?"

And I said, "Well, it's invasive, poorly differentiated, ductal adeno-carcinoma grade 2 (nuclear grade 2 out of 3) 1.2 centimeters."

Allen replied loudly, "Oh. Okay. Well, if so, you only need a lumpectomy. I mean, who would ever, in this day and age, do a mastectomy on something like this. 1.2 centimeters...That's a tiny thing. That's early detection. You don't even have to worry about who does the surgery. It's a piece of cake for any surgeon," he says. "Afterwards, with the pathology report, you need to be a little smart to know what to do next but right now, <u>nothing</u>. Research has shown the survival rate, which <u>means living without recurrence</u> (it doesn't just mean surviving) is the same for mastectomy and lumpectomy. And, when you've got your pathology report, come on over to Atlanta, have a good time here and stop in and see me. I'll be happy to review your report."

Oh—we could even have a good time! Oh! What a wonderful thought.

We put the phone down and just looked at each other. And we said, "This guy has just given us a treasure! <u>We are in charge</u> of this thing. And we are going to go find a team that inspires us, the way this man inspired us, to know just exactly what we want to do, how we want to do it, with whom we want to do it, and so on." So we both sort of straightened our bodies up, you know, and looked at each other and the first thing we did is we called the plastic surgeon to cancel our appointment! We are not interested in plastic surgery, and we are not even interested in finding out about plastic surgery. We are going to search for a dream team.

## We're in Charge Here!

*"This guy has just given us a treasure!*
*We are in charge of this thing.*
*And we are going to find a team*
*that inspires us, the way this man*
*has inspired us, to know just exactly*
*what we want to do, how we want to do it,*
*with whom we want to do it, and so on...*
*We are going to search for a dream team."*

# Chapter 4

# The Search for "The Boob Dream Team"

*Hedy promptly began sampling the smorgasbord of medical and surgical options, one interview at a time. It was obvious that the Kosher Choreographer was still very busy orchestrating the flow of options. It was also clear that it was as important that the doctors be exposed to her passionate, inspired tenaciousness for the human connection, as it was for her to hear what they had to offer medically and surgically. The exchange subtly reminded each of them, one by one, of who they really were as human beings. Her passion for connecting with the human spirit and magnifying the best, undoubtedly drew out the best in them. There's a good chance that it even reminded them of the reason they originally wanted to become a physician...something that had perhaps dimmed during daily chaos and stress. There's nothing like that feeling of knowing that you truly enhanced another human being on a profound level. There's nothing like the feeling that you are tapped into your Authentic Self. One way or another, this connection of human spirit was a basic requirement for Hedy. None would soon forget her visit.*

So that day, we began to call around. We cancelled the appointment with the plastic surgeon but decided to keep another appointment with the radiation oncologist, that my friend had set up. We kept that one because we thought, "You know what?

We want to find out about radiation oncology." At the end of the day, we looked at each other and we said, "Wasn't this a gorgeous day?" (It was a gorgeous day!) We did what we wanted to do. We went to Timothy's Gallery and exchanged something. And we shopped for a bra because I'm going to need to wear soft bras. We just sort of took the day to integrate the news.

Then, off we went to the radiation oncologist. It turned out to be a gorgeous place. People refer to it as the Taj Mahal. *[louder and emphatically]:* A gorgeous, gorgeous place—BUT, *[continuing in a staccato-monotone]:* we went in and quickly noticed that there wasn't a "welcome." There was a sign-in sheet and the usual bunch of papers to fill out. The place is beautiful and there's coffee and good cookies. They had hot chocolate and tea. But no one welcomed you. I said to Yumi, "There has to be a welcome for everybody that comes through this door... especially in a cancer center!"

Then this black woman arrives with her little girl. And it's hard to know why these two would be in a cancer center. I wondered, "What is it? Is the little child sick with cancer? Is the mother sick with cancer? What is going on?" I am so curious about everything. So, we began to wait. Everywhere you wait. But, I decided I didn't want to just "wait." This is my life right now. And, instead of just waiting, I want to get to know this wonderful black woman with her little child. So I went over.

"This is your child?" She said, "Yes, it is."

"What is her name?" She said, "Tatyana."

"Oh, that's a Russian name!" She said, "I know. I wanted to give her a Russian name."

"How old is she?" She replied, "Four months old."

"Oh, can I hold her? My granddaughter is a week old and I was going to go see her in Israel, but now I have to see the doctor instead."

She said, "Of course, you can hold her."

So, I'm holding this adorable little Tatyana. I looked at her... and she looked at me. And Judie, she began to talk to me! And, I answer her in jibberish... "Poo pooit to." And we have this conversation back and forth! And the mother says, "She's never talked like this. I can't believe what's happening here." I said, "Really?" Well, Tatyana and I had this most profound conversation and then she began to <u>smile</u> at me. I couldn't help but smile back. Her mother said, "She has never smiled like this." I said, "I don't know what's happening. Maybe she knows I'm a little scared today, and she's trying to soothe me." And we continued to chat for awhile.

*Nothing like being swept up in the pure, loving tones of an infant to settle us down inside and "reconnect" us! What a rich exchange!*

The entire visit was so soothing and just what I needed. Eventually I said to the mother, "Why are <u>you</u> here?" And she showed me her ear. Well, it turns out that she had a cancerous growth around her ear. She said that the growth can be cut off, but if radiation isn't performed after the surgery, it comes back. So she showed me the stitches and she said, "I'm getting radiation and then they'll take out the stitches. It's going to be okay." And I said, "That's wonderful!"

*There's waiting...and then there's "quality waiting."*

It was a wonderful visit and a rich experience. We were interrupted when the nurse suddenly called my name and promptly took me to a scale to be weighed. Do you know how many times I've been weighed lately? Every time you go to a doctor they weigh you. And on the history that accompanies the pathology report I am routinely described as "a slightly overweight female." I said to Yumi, "I have my identity! *[laughing uncontrollably]:* I'm a slightly overweight female!" So they checked my weight everywhere I went, and found out that I'm still a slightly overweight female. It was unbelievable. Everywhere I was, they weighed me. I thought, why are they weighing me? I just want to talk to this man. I want to see if he's the one for me!

Then they promptly took me into this examining room, and I said to the nurse, *[softly]:* "Is there someplace else I can talk to the doctor?"

And she said, "No. This is where the doctor sees patients."

I said, "But I'm not going to be examined. I just want to talk to him."

"This is where he talks to people."

I said, "I see."

Well, he comes in, and you know—you've seen it before—he picks up your chart and comes in, kind of looks at you—but, kind-of-doesn't look because he doesn't really have to. All the data about you is in the chart.

So he begins, "Hello. What brings you here today?" I said, "Doctor, I'd like to not talk to you in here."

"Oh, but this is where I talk to people." I said, "I know. Your nurse told me, but I must talk to you in a conference room."

"Well, but this is where I see all my patients."

I said, "But, Doctor, I'm not your patient yet. I'm Hedy Schleifer, and I haven't chosen to be a patient yet. I may choose to become one, but I'm not one yet, and I must talk to you as Hedy Schleifer."

*Perfect.* **Perfect. Perfect!**

He says, "But I don't have another suitable place." (Now this is the Taj Mahal, and spans two floors!)

I said, "Let's go find one."

To his credit, he agreed. He said, "Okay, but in all my years as a doctor this has never been necessary."

*[with glee]: Uh huh! Fabulous!*

So we go traipsing around this man's office. He is one of four partners who own this center, and he can't find a place to sit where he can just talk, like you and I are talking right now. But

## Not So Fast, Doctor!
### (after being shown to an exam room)

...*"But, Doctor, I'd like to talk to you
in a conference room."*

*He said, "But this is where I see all my patients."*

*"But Doctor, I'm Hedy Schleifer,
and I haven't chosen to become a patient yet!...
I must talk to you as Hedy Schleifer!"*

*He said, "But I don't have a suitable place."*

*I said, "Then let's go find one."*

to his credit, he traipsed around—the nurses were watching this doctor and the two people behind him, walking through the center looking for a place to sit. One place after another was unsuitable—his office was a mess and couldn't be used—another room wasn't appropriate—here's a place but not enough chairs. Finally, he finds a place! So we sit, and begin once again.

And he says, "Okay, okay. What can I do for you...what is it that you want?" And I said, warmly, "Relax. I have never had a radiation oncologist before. I'm a virgin. You're my first!" (He softened a little.) "You're the first and I want to hear everything you have to say about radiation oncology."

Well, he began at first a bit defensively. Slowly but surely, with our questions, he really began to tell us what radiation is and what are some of the side effects, and why it's been done, and what other illnesses it's being done for, and his own training, and he just kept talking and talking and talking and he just completely relaxed. Yumi had written a lot of questions and we asked them all. When we were done, I said, "Now what is the question we haven't asked...the question that you would want your sister to ask a radiation oncologist?"

*Perfect.*

# The Leading Question

*"Now, what is the question we haven't asked...*
*the question that you would want your sister*
*to ask a radiation oncologist?"*

He said, "Oh well, I would want her to know how people are going to treat her and what's going to happen and to see the machine." And I said, "Oh, I want to do all that." He said, "Okay."

Well, he just couldn't let us leave. An hour-and-a-half later he was still talking to us. The waiting room was full. Finally, we needed to go because we had a workshop to prepare for. So we got up and he followed us saying, "And do you have children?" and "How old are they?" and "Oh, you're a grandmother?" He just couldn't stop, and he walked us to the door of the center.

*You blew his cover! What a profound vision. The three of you, serpentine-ing through the corridors, being led by inspiration. Winding through this hallway and that, and on an invisible energetic level, simultaneously stirrrrr-ing all that was previously thought to be "normal protocol." You paraded around with such a simple mission, to obtain a proper place to speak as one human being to another and as equals. You could just feel him begin to pull off the protective layering that was covering his Authentic Self: The one who chose to be a physician because he cared about people, the one who truly wanted to be of great help, the one who wanted to facilitate healing in others, the one who wasn't afraid to deeply connect with patients, the one who was energetic and eager to reach as many people with his skills, talent and compassion as possible, the one who felt fabulously alive and so pleased to be a physician. He's ba-ack!*

Indeed, he's **back!** *[softly]:* I wrote him a beautiful letter.

You know, becoming a patient is a decision, not an automatic thing. It's a decision that you make, over and over again. In this culture, it seems to be taken for granted upon your arrival, that you are suddenly a patient. But I must be in charge of this decision, before I will surrender to their expertise. Each would have to inspire me on three levels: as a person, a scientist and a professional.

---

## *Decision versus Assumption!*

*You know, becoming a patient is a decision,*
*not an automatic thing.*
*It's a decision that you make, over and over again.*
*In this culture, it seems*
*to be taken for granted upon your arrival,*
*that you are suddenly a patient.*

*But, I must be in charge of this decision,*
*before I will surrender to their expertise.*

*Each doctor would have to inspire me on three levels:*
*as a person, a scientist and a professional.*

---

The next day was Friday, and the day before our couple's workshop in Ft. Lauderdale on "Getting The Love You Want." Seventeen couples were registered and we made a decision that we were still going to do the workshop. We said, "Not only are we going to do the workshop, we won't tell them about this until the end, because otherwise they'd focus on us." The couples are very vulnerable during the weekend and we need to be centered... so we will tell them at the end. And we also said, "Enough discussion about cancer." We made the decision and put it away. Now, it didn't stay away. Occasionally it came knocking at our door. But every time it knocked at the door, we said, *[melodically]*: "Sor-ry. ♪♪ We can't let you in right now because we have a workshop to do!" *[laughing]*

*Behavioral modification for cancer! YOU tell cancer it'll have to wait...it knocks intermittently...in vain.*

And, *[in a near whisper]:* I said to Yumi, "These workshops are not only our mission in life, but the sacredness in each gathering reaches back and repeatedly touches us both." This particular one was timed perfectly in our journey because it drew upon our steadiness and our spiritual connection. It pulled these qualities through us more than ever before. We always love setting up the room because we think about every couple. We bless the manuals as we place them around the room. I mean, our ritual of setting up the room, was and is, the very best thing for us. We put music on and we dance around the room. We fill the room with a blessing and an energetic welcome. As a result, the couples just feel totally at ease; they relax, and they just do amazing work. Preparing the room is crucial for the participants' best possible experience. This time it was clear that it was crucial for our experience as well.

*The two of you set the stage with an invisible blessing that ultimately "gets all over you, and all through you" at the same time! Rather like the gift that keeps on giving.*

Absolutely. Invisible and profound. And the room just becomes so sacred. And then, of course, we always have our Sabbath ceremony in our hotel room with the singing and the praying and the lighting of the candles that are a part of that. And we think of the couples and bless them and we ask God to bless us. And—it's just this wonderful ceremony we have. It's very centering.

## The Lumpectomy Dance

So Saturday morning before a workshop I woke up inspired to dance the Lumpectomy Dance. Do you know about the Lumpectomy Dance?

*Not yet! You gonna show me?*

I don't quite remember the melody. But it's like this. I was just dancing it with the melody and I was dancing all around *[illustrating in my kitchen]:* singing:

> "Choon-kee ♪♪ choon-kee, ♪♪
>
> Out with you. ♪♪
>
> Just you,
>
> Out with just you!
>
> Around you is cleaner,
>
> Around you is clean.
>
> Choon-kee, choon-kee, ♪♪
>
> Out with you.
>
> Also from here,
>
> A little bit out,
>
> Confirming that the node is negative,
>
> That we took out!"
>
> *[laughter]*

I was just dancing this dance, naked!

*You almost left out the naked part!*

Yes...yes, I was naked! I danced it naked and I just kind of, you know, got this thing out, and cleaned it all up to music and dance. Then I called Yumi and I said, *[with a shy, flirtatious grin]:* "I've been practicing the Lumpectomy Dance. Would you like to see it? It's like the Macarena, but different!" *[laughing]*

So, I just danced and sang. I did it because I really wanted to be centered for the workshop. I felt that if I didn't, you know, make friends with the lumpectomy in advance, it would have interfered. So I danced the Lumpectomy Dance! And I sang, and I danced some more.

*You celebrated the experience in advance of the surgery—and aligned yourself with the event instead of resisting and dreading it. Instead of losing Life Force, you reclaimed your power—and danced your way into alignment! Wow!*

Exactly. It absolutely neutralized my thoughts around my upcoming surgery.

So we went into this workshop and, yes, the issue we were dealing with was knocking at the door, but ever so slightly. We did the workshop. Judie, *[softly and with eyes of wonder]:* we were more powerful than we've ever been. **<u>Ever</u>**! I mean, *[boldly and loudly]:* our message about commitment *[pounding hand on table with each attribute]:* and love and unconditional giving and all the things that we talk about were not only assimilated faster with this group, but the entire group seemed to reach a whole new level. These people did phenomenal work. And at the end of the workshop, we said, "You know, this is the first workshop in which we are sharing something new and very personal with the couples. We've just gotten this diagnosis. This is a challenge we're facing..." and we explained the situation. Then we asked the couples if there was anything they wanted to say, and people had wonderful wishes and prayers and so forth.

We always say goodbye to every couple as they leave the workshop. *[softly whispering]:* This one couple came past to say goodbye, and the gentleman says, "You know, I'm a plastic surgeon. I live in Vero Beach. I have a friend who's not only an oncologist, but she had breast cancer three-and-a-half years ago. I feel that you and she must meet. You just have to meet." The interesting thing is that we had to be in Vero Beach the following day because that's where Yumi's business is. We were already going to go to Vero Beach whether we needed to meet this woman or not! Were we meant to be there? I mean, look at this!

*Perfect.*

That night we stayed with Yumi's father. Do you know about Yumi's father? He's 97 years old. He looks as young as you and me, and he lives like you and me. He cooks and he cleans, and he does laundry, and he helps his neighbors. He grieved for his wife of 72 years, and then he started a new life. We adore him. So we went to visit him and told him that I was going to have an operation. We didn't tell him the whole story, but we told him a little of it, and that he needs to begin to pray for me, because he's such a good pray-er. He's just so glad to offer his prayers, and we're so grateful to have them.

## *The Sentinel Node is Calling*

The next morning, we left for Vero Beach and went directly to see our friend, the plastic surgeon. He dropped everything. Judie, he dropped everything! He said goodbye to his staff and personally took us to his oncologist friend. It was as if all he had to do was welcome Yumi and Hedy and take them to this friend.

We found her a very interesting woman. She's German, slim, blonde, a very professional European doctor. We were absolutely delighted when she showed us into this wonderful conference room, so that we could talk. What a pleasure! A room that was set up to be used for conferences! And then she said, "Let me tell you my story."

Well, her story was that when she discovered she had breast cancer, she decided to have a mastectomy. She decided to have a mastectomy because *[pounding on table for emphasis]:* she – had – no – time – for – anything – else! She wanted her breast off, *[slapping hands together]:* and to get back to work! I thought, "This is not for me, but that is what she wanted." Powerful! She basically said, "This is what I chose to do, and I'm doing very well, and da-da-da-da-da-da-dah."…"And Hedy," she said, "don't be special. Be a <u>patient</u>. Just go someplace where they don't know you, so you can just be a patient. Why did God want me to have this? You know what? God wanted me to have this experience so that I can be a much better doctor because I now know from inside out what it's like to be a patient." She continued, "And, be sure to read *Close to the Bone,* a wonderful book on spirituality by Dr. Jean Shinoda Bolen." "And," she said, "find out about the sentinel node."[2] (Now this last statement is what got my attention! This part of the conversation was an absolute gift! Ding, ding!) I said, "O-o-o-oh, the sentinel node. What is that?" She said, "Well, it's new." And she began to explain a little bit about it. Something inside me stirred as I heard about the sentinel node. I tucked it in my memory for future reference. I knew that I wanted to learn more about the sentinel node.

On Tuesday we had an appointment with another surgeon who was also referred by my gynecologist. During the visit, I said, "You mentioned something on the phone about breast mapping. What is that?"

"Well," she said, "We don't actually do breast mapping."

I said, "Well, but what is it?"

"Well, there are some centers, very few, who actually do it. It's a process which allows you to actually locate the sentinel node."

*[As if she is a private investigator who has secretly latched on to a critical piece in a puzzle]:* "Oh, it does, does it? But, you don't really do it here yet?"

"No. No, we don't."

Okay. Meanwhile, she performed a biopsy on the tiny cyst on my opposite breast, which we later found out was benign. I said, "You know, this breast mapping and sentinel node thing has been brought to my attention over and over again. I am very interested in it."

She said, "Oh, Hedy, you don't want that. You are much too special for that." (Think of that.) She continued with what amounted to, "It's leading-edge research that allows people to avoid being cut open, but doctors are used to doing the other way. I'd rather take all your nodes out. You are much too special to only have one node taken out. You should have all the nodes taken out. Whether you need it or not!"

*So you can reeeeaaaaally be special!*

You know I'm being facetious, but isn't that amazing! And this is a splendid doctor...a splendid doctor. I felt like saying, "Well, I know I'm special, but I am going to find out about this sentinel node!"

# Chapter 5

# Soul Food

It seemed as if there were appointments to keep every single day. From the beginning, we began a ritual of following a day of medical appointments with something special and fun. Every single day we went to a special place or did something that was nurturing. This time, after that biopsy, we went to a little gathering of dear friends.

*It's so easy to lose your "self" while you are actively involved in the medical system, not to mention sporting a new diagnosis. There's so much there that can potentially short-circuit your peace of mind and well-being. So much unfamiliar territory, so many rules…you are continually being molded into compliance with this routine and that, with this schedule and more of that. It can, unless you are careful, put "Joy" on hold. What a wonderful antidote "fun" is for whatever each day held. What a wonderful daily touchstone! It's like, after all is said and done (and poked and scoped), "I'm going to celebrate the truth of who I am and celebrate life itself! I'm going to touch what is truly real! Oooh, let me hug another friend!"*

Yes, celebrating what's "real" has absolutely become our "soul food" in each day.

On the Monday after we came back from Vero Beach, we went out to our favorite little coffee shop on Park Avenue. I go there often and take my work with me. They have little tables where I like to write. There's a young man named David who works there and he always says hello. We've had profound talks. You know, while I'm having my cup of coffee and writing letters, we've had these wonderfully profound chats.

So when we arrived, we were delighted to find that David was our waiter. As he came to our table, I said, "David, I just want to tell you—I'm struggling with what to do. I've had a diagnosis of cancer in my breast, and I'm not yet sure, you know, who's going to do what and how it's going to be, but I'm working on it." "Oh," he said (a pondering sort of "Oh"). He went away; then he came back and said, "Hedy, you know that this thing has nothing to do with who you are today. This is something old that just has to be taken out."

I said to Yumi, "You know, he's right. This has nothing to do with life today. It just has to be taken out." It was amazing. David returned again and said, "Hedy, I used to be part of a group that was working with a guru named *[playfully making up words]:* Mama Baya Baba. Whatever! I don't remember the name."

*Baba someone!*

It was a Baba. *[laughing]* He told of a certain woman who followed this Baba and his teachings. Anyway, he says, "One day before the guru's talk to all of his disciples, the woman was sitting in the office and a picture of the Baba fell off the wall. As she picked it up, she found these words written on the back.

'Everything is

## all

right.'

'All' was a separate word."

So David says to me, "I just want you to know, everything is **all** right."

*All is well.*

Yes! All is well. And he left again. You know, he had work to do. But every time he returned, he was like a perfect Elijah, a prophet leaving words of wisdom. Yumi and I just looked at each other.

*A perfect Elijah coming to the table in the guise of a waiter giving you a message.*

It was just so clear. He said, "This has got nothing to do with you today. It's an old thing. It's got to come out and everything is **all** right." That's how that strikes me.

Yumi said, "You know, you are amazing. Every place you go, there is that soul connection that you've previously made with a person who now nurtures you in return."

What a surprise. I mean, I never knew that this wonderful young man was really someone who had been involved with all this other…being with the Babas and all of that. And here he was in my life once again, like many other times, but this time playing the part of—

*An angel in disguise?*

Yes! That's it! A wonderful divine messenger. I've always known that he was a very, very special soul but I've never known this other part of him. I go for coffee and he includes two profound messages!

*And all for the price of one, even though the messages are priceless!*

Priceless! Yumi and I just cried.

So the next day I e-mailed a note to all of the therapists who had heard about my diagnosis. In it I said, "I've turned a corner. I now know this is nothing to do with who I am today. But, it's got to get out of there. And everything is **all** right!"

*Imagine what the cells in your body are doing at that time? Imagine what they're doing when you take in the thought that*

*"everything is all right" or "all is well." My personal vision for
those moments is a wild cellular celebration choreographed by
Life Force. Cells throughout your body simultaneously hooting,
hollering, giggling, and dancing. What a powerful "now."*

Yes. The body just relaxes into its best. It feels wonderful.

*You know, any time we embrace the truth that "all is well," we are
in perfect alignment to receive the next magical moment—and the
next and the next. But the first step always lies in finding a way
to begin to feel good. Appreciation is the easiest and surest way
to start feeling good. And you, Hedy, are sooo good at appreciating. I'd say you're a professional appreciate-or! We should have
some new business cards made up for you! You appreciate in every
direction and find the magic that's hidden in the drama of every-
day life: in conversations, scenery, books, music, food, clothing,
jewelry, art, relationships, medical offices, hospitals, and coffee
shops on Park Avenue! Appreciation and "generic joy" (joy about
anything!) are sacred siphons that pull in more of all that we
consider wonderful and magical.*

I love that…"Generic Joy!" Jumping for "Generic Joy!" *[laugh-
ing]* Feeling good for any reason.

 *Jumping for Generic Joy!*

*You know, any time we embrace the truth that
"all is well" we are in perfect alignment to receive the
next magical moment—and the next and the next.
But the first step always lies in finding a way to feel good.
Appreciation is the easiest and surest way to start
feeling good. Appreciation and "generic joy" (joy about
anything!) are sacred siphons that pull in more of
all that we consider wonderful and magical.*

*For any reason whatsoever! Your cells don't care what you're feeling good about—they thrive on any joyful occasion. They look for any opportunity, any reason, to go for a joy-ride! "Generic Joy" unleashes the Life Force in each cell. It instantly dissolves barriers where energy was previously stuck. The perfect antidote for all ailments!*

## Disowning a Disease

### *(Here...you take it! I don't want it!...*
### *You take it! It's not mine!*
### *I'm busy celebrating this fabulous body of mine!)*

Well, the next day we found ourselves in the waiting room at the surgeon's office. We waited and we waited and we waited! And, when we finally got in there, I was weighed once again! *[laughing]* I mean, hey! And I was put in this teeny, tiny examining room. And I said to the nurse, "You know, I just want to talk to the surgeon. Is there another place?" And she said, "No. This is where the doctor talks to patients." I thought, "Well, I know how to handle this."

It went something like this...The doctor came into the teeny, tiny room. He appeared to have a very rigid demeanor and was very business-like. He did not make eye contact with us at all. His first words were, "Where are your mammograms? I need to see your mammograms." I said, "I'll give them to you in a second, but first I'd like to talk to you."

He replied briskly, "I don't talk. I'm a surgeon."

I said, "Well, with me you have to talk because I can't do anything before we look into each other's eyes and we talk some."

"If you want a person who talks, then you're not in the right place."

And Yumi says, "Well, for a patient to relax they need to know that they have a comfortable relationship with their doctor."

He said (curtly and impatiently), "That's not what I'm into. I'm an excellent surgeon. Surgery is what I do. I don't do talking.

(raising his voice) I have been in practice for a very long time and this is the first time this has happened to me. People come to me for the excellent work I do. I have made a special appointment to work you into my schedule here today, and quite frankly **I don't need this kind of stuff.**"

I began softly, "Well, you know, everybody that meets me has a first time experience." With this, he immediately looked up. Slowly and deliberately, I said, "Doctor, I'm very uncomfortable. My heart is pounding, I am sweating, I am sitting here having lots and lots of very uncomfortable feelings, and yet I do want to talk to you. So let us pretend that you've just come into the room and if there's no other place we can talk, let's talk here, but let's talk."

He said, "Okay. What do you want to talk about?"

I said, "I want to talk about the sentinel node."

That instantly got his attention. Eyes fixed on mine, and sitting a bit straighter, he said, "What do you know about it?"

I said, "Well, I know very little about it. I just know that there's something called breast mapping with the injection of dye and radioactive material. I know that there is the possibility of finding the sentinel node. I want to know everything about it."

He said (increasing in excitement), "Well, as a matter of fact, I'm one who is currently trying to bring this to Orlando. I am very excited about this possibility," he said. "You know, women have had to have surgery and haven't had options like this one, until now." (I mean, this man is really a good man. But he just has forgotten how to be with people. He is so excited that women will have this option, but he doesn't know how to do the procedure well enough yet. He's still being trained.) He went on saying that he's studying with the people in Sarasota.

I said, "Oh, the people in Sarasota. Who are they? What are they doing?"

He said, "They have been pioneering this technique and they've already done about 200 women and they—(he paused)— Let me call them and tell them about you and maybe we can arrange an appointment for you there. They can tell you all about it, and you can see the center at the same time."

This same man who wouldn't even look at me in the beginning, had transformed into an energized, enthused, compassionate man who couldn't do enough for us. He talked for about an hour about why this new procedure is so good, and why this is so important, and why he wants to bring it to Orlando, and how tough it is, and politically, and what it will mean for this area... and, I mean, he just shared himself. He also called the people in Sarasota and made an appointment for us the following Monday, even though it's normally impossible to get in so quickly. It usually takes a month to just get an appointment. The appointment would be with a physician named Dr. Robert Walker who does the research on breasts.

Returning from making the appointment, he said, "This is very exciting. After you see them, if you want me to follow you as your doctor, I'll be glad to be your doctor. Or, if you want them to follow you through this, that's fine. Just do whatever you think is right." He continued, "This lesion is in a place that's fairly rare. It would be such a marvelous addition to the work they're doing."

He went on about this and that. It was like he was "in heaven." And, like the other physician, he couldn't leave us either. We were with him for an hour and fifteen minutes. As we were leaving, he took my hand and said, "I would like to apologize for the way that I behaved in the beginning of our time together." He said, "You know, I'm a blockhead."

I said, "You know what? You are a blockhead, yes, you are! But you are also a really courageous doctor with vision and compassion, and I thank you!" As we came out, his waiting room was full.

*You must admit that he was also "full" of elation. He was full of himself, his Authentic Self!*

Absolutely. It was a very rich exchange.

*Once again, here's another person who "reconnected" with their*

*"Authentic Self" during a visit with you. It's like a cram course in "Back to Basics." (even for blockheads!) Back to remembering the deliciousness of human spirit, and it's as simple as establishing eye contact and speaking from the heart. You re-awakened his better nature, his Authentic Self! Think of all the patients that saw him afterwards who benefited by that exchange. Whether they knew it or not, it was worth their delay in the waiting room!*

Yes, one blockhead now all fluffed up!

He also got us another appointment that same day with the radiation oncologist who works with him. So we went on to that appointment. On one level, everything went very well with this one. You know, we were able to talk first and then I was examined. It went very well! I mean, he was so willing to meet my needs. I think he had been warned!

*Tipped off! [chuckling]*

Yes, tipped off. So we had a talk and then he examined me, and then I got dressed again, and then we had our discussion.

*[simultaneously]: The word is out! [laughing]*

I said, "Tell me everything about radiation." And he did, and he was very kind. At first, he was like an old-fashioned family doctor. You know that wonderful feeling you have? Very present, very sweet, and very nice. I want to write him a letter about that. But I also want to write the letter about what I'm going to tell you next.

At some point he said, "You know, the reason we want to do the radiation is because your cancer..."

I said, "Stop it right there, Doctor." I said, "It is not <u>my cancer</u>. It is a <u>diagnosis</u> of cancer." (Which is so funny. You know, I hadn't gotten your letter yet. It was amazing to find this same thing in your letter.) I said to him, "How can I use my energy to try to own this thing, and try to get rid of it, at the same time?"

*Oh, perfect! [squealing]*

I said to him, "It neutralizes the whole thing. I am not going to use my energy to get rid of it." I said, "I'm going to use my energy to own what is really mine, this phenomenal body." He sat there, a bit offset, and proceeded to go right down another track—and it wasn't the track I'm on. I gradually realized that he had a spiel. So, on one level, we had an appropriate setting with time allotted to talk, but on another level, it wasn't really what I was looking for. He didn't really talk to me. He talked to all women in general who have, or have had, a diagnosis of cancer. I got him off track from his spiel, so he just said a few more things and said, "And that's about it." And I said, "Well, thank you and you're a very kind person." He really is just a kind, good person.

---

## Halt! Don't Go There!

The doctor said, "In the case of your cancer..."
I said, "Stop right there, Doctor! It is not my cancer.
It is a diagnosis of cancer."

"How can I use my energy to try to own this thing
and try to get rid of it at the same time?
It neutralizes the whole thing. I'm not going to use my
energy to get rid of it... I'm going to use my energy to
own what is really mine, this phenomenal body!"

---

So then we went to the waiting room to wait for the nurse who sort of coordinates things for them. Yumi said, "Where do you want to sit?" I said, "You see over there? It's for the little children. They have these little chairs. Let's go there! Let's just go sit on those little chairs." So we sat in these little chairs. And lo and behold, Judie, on the floor was a stack of books. One of the books was titled, *My Radiation Therapy Day*[1] for children with cancer. As I read through it, I said, "This is the way all of us need to be spoken to." It talked about radiation being like a radio...ther-apy, radio-ther-apy. The book is so lovely. I asked if I could take this book because that's going to be my book. If I'm going to need radiation therapy, I want that to be my accompaniment. Not any of the stuff I'm getting in these little booklets that scare you. This is just about your soul, and about your friends, and about what you need, and about your feelings, and about, you know, what might scare you, and so on.

The coordinator said I could have the book and that, "Anytime you need anything just do it through me." And if we had gone with that team, she would have been a wonderful person to work with. But you know what? I wasn't inspired. I wasn't inspired by the surgeon and I wasn't inspired by the radiation oncologist. I knew that I would not choose them to be on my team.

## *The Missing Link— Inspiration*

*But you know what? I wasn't inspired.
I wasn't inspired by the surgeon and
I wasn't inspired
by the radiation oncologist.
I knew that I would not
choose them to be on my team.*

*Just remember that there's a very good chance that you left him with a gift of seeing through new eyes. That it is not your cancer, you're not owning it...you're owning your phenomenal body. Imagine what a gift that was. It's as if you're just leaving this long trail—*

Yes, I'm leaving a trail. And now I'm writing to all of them so they're going to have it in writing. You know, I'm also leaving a paper trail!

# Searching for Your Soul in the CAT Scan Unit!

So that was Wednesday. And on Thursday I had a tough day; and the reason it was tough is because they sent me for a pre-operative bone scan,[2] CAT scan[3] of the stomach, and chest x-ray, all on the same day. I went to the hospital feeling strong and wonderful. I came out of that hospital five hours later, thoroughly exhausted. At times, the atmosphere actually felt toxic.

*Invisible energy that can take it's toll on the human spirit...if you're unprepared for it. Imagine, in just the past month, all the other people that were in the same CAT scan unit before you, who were absolutely terrified. The CAT scan unit is energetically loaded with invisible leftovers from the experiences of others. Things like fear, "What if's," "What's that's," vulnerability, and powerlessness.*

Everywhere!

*I love to intentionally fill any anticipated environment with good things before I even leave for the appointment, and while I'm actually there. You can, for example, easily (intentionally) fill the waiting rooms, the CAT scan unit, and x-ray department, etc., with the energy of "all is well." You merely hold that thought as you reference those areas. You only need to do it for a little over a minute for each area. (Or do them as a collective group.) Energetically touch those who will be working with you during the tests with the vision of them tapping into their original passion for becoming health professionals. Anticipate a thoughtful hospital staff, and interesting patients you will meet as you wait together, etc. You don't have to take my word for it. You've already experienced the toll that a day of disconnection can take on you. Try playing this visual (invisible) game first and see the difference it makes! Then show up for the tests, eager to see evidence of these same wonderful things and more.*

You're right. I've already experienced the unpleasant version. I'm ready to have a better experience next time. I hadn't thought of doing something like you've suggested prior to the appointment.

*My favorite technique is to (in my mind's eye) visualize this person as they were at three months old. Then I put them over my shoulder and rock them in my mind while saying, "Remember who you are," or "All is well." It means I am joining the vision of them in full spiritual connection. It means I am joining the vision of them fully tapped into their spiritual guidance and making good decisions. I have energetically joined their Authentic Self by focusing on their innocence, or who they were before experiencing things that closed them down. A three-month-old seems to be the perfect touchstone for this. It's a quick and easy way to energetically massage their true nature—and mine! The real gift is that I'm simultaneously feeling my spiritual connection.*

*So, on a day filled with appointments, you could for example, spend all that spare time (in the waiting areas, etc.) rocking everyone you see. Generically rock everyone who has ever been in that CAT scan unit before you (people you'll never meet), as well as those who will find themselves inside it in the future. It energetically sets the tone for you <u>and</u> others who follow, as well. (Another gift that keeps on giving!) Just as you can't "own cancer"*

## Rocking
### ...perfect for those helpless moments
### ...perfect for "Waiting"

My favorite technique is to visualize this person as they were at three months old. Then I put them over my shoulder and rock them in my mind while saying, "Remember who you are," or "All is well." It means I am joining the vision of them in full spiritual connection. It's a quick and easy way to energetically massage their true nature—and mine! The real gift is that I'm feeling my spiritual connection simultaneously.

*and "get rid of it" at the same time, you can't use your energy for setting a positive tone, and fight what you call "toxic energy" at the same time. One cancels the other. You might as well choose the one that feels wonderful—one that makes a positive difference in your experience. It's easy, fast, free, portable, and a great way to pass time while you are waiting. It's a way of having an entirely different experience while going for the same tests you had, and yet returning home feeling strong and vibrant.*

That's such a fabulous thought. This experience was so exhausting. I'm ready to have it be the last one of its kind!

*Sure it was. If you could go into rewind and do it again, deliberately choosing thoughts and visions that feel good (before, during and after), it would truly give you the advantage. It's a good thing to remember to do for all "tours de test" in medical environments. Otherwise, the conscious or unconscious awareness of the negative energy can suck you dry.*

It really did. I'd much rather have surfaced at the end of the day feeling strong and wonderful.

## *Breaking the Rules...*
## *Illuminating the Spirit*

Oh, I must tell you that the week before this, we had a very interesting event. Prior to my diagnosis, I was having menopausal symptoms and my heart was doing all these funny things. Just to be safe, I had been scheduled for a stress EKG (cardiogram). It turned out that the stress EKG actually took place the week after the diagnosis. The test went well, and my heart is fantastically strong, but we had to check it out. So I went to the clinic, where they would do this test. It is not a hospital, it's a private clinic. And when we arrived at the clinic where the stress EKG would be done, the young woman, Kathleen, says to Yumi very sweetly, "Sir, you'll have to wait here."

Softy, I said, "And why is that?"

She says, "Well, because that's how it is, you know, the patient comes in and the partner stays there."

I said, sweetly, "Why?" She says, "Because, you know, this is the place where they do the testing and the doctor is here for the patient—but <u>not</u> the partner."

Again, I said, "Why?"

She says, "Well, because it's the rule."

I said, "Why? Why?"

She said, "I don't know!" laughing.

I said warmly and delighting in this, "Kathleen, let's break the rule!"

She said, "Really?"

I said, "Yes. Today we break the rule! My husband comes in! Because, you know, he is really my partner and he is my friend. And, whatever I do with him around is so much better. We support each other, and we love each other so much, and we don't want to be separated. Especially not during a time like this."

She said, "That makes a lot of sense."

So Yumi was allowed in, and was at my side when the doctor came in. I said (with a smile), "Doctor, Kathleen broke the rule!" And she started to laugh. And I said, "Yes, she told us it was the rule, but she broke the rule." I said, "You must be having a lot of trouble with Kathleen because she must be breaking the rules all over the place."

And Kathleen started to laugh, and she says, "Yes, and I want to break this rule again!"

Anyway, Yumi was there and it was just wonderful together.

As we left, Kathleen came over with this radiant face, looking so lovely. She said we had absolutely liberated her. She said, "Thank you for what you've shown me. The importance of the loving partner being right there with their partner. I will never forget the two of you, and I will never forget your relationship, and I will never forget this afternoon."

Well, with that in tow, we arrived there in the hospital for those three tests. And the first thing was the stomach scan, you

# "Togetherness" versus "The Rules"

*(Yumi was allowed to
break the rules and stay with me.)
The young woman said, "Thank you for
what you've shown me...the importance of the
loving partner being right there with their partner.*

*I will never forget the two of you, and
I will never forget your relationship,
and I will never forget this afternoon."*

know, that big room and that machine and you know, that whole thing. And I said to the woman, "Can my husband be there with me?" And she said, "Oh, no. I'm so sorry. He can't." I said, "Why?" (Here we go again!) And she said, "Well, because it's dangerous. It's radiation." I said softly, "Do you have an apron that he could wear?" She said, "Yes." I said, "Well, then can he be in there if he wears a protective apron?" She says, "Well, I don't see why not."

I said, "Thank you. It's very important. He must be there. He is my lover and my friend and he must be with me."

To my delight, Yumi was allowed to join me. He checked with her to see whether he could stand close to me, and whether he could touch me.

She said, "I don't see why not."

So while this thing was going on, he was touching my forehead. I began to cry as he was caressing me.

She said, "Oh, she is so scared. She has got so much on her mind." And Yumi said, "She's not crying because of that. She's crying because she feels attended to and loved."

And I said, "That's right. I'm crying because I feel attended to, and I feel loved, and I feel so happy."

And the woman said, "What a refreshing way to look at this. His presence makes you happy. Oh."

Isn't that something? It's like so-o-o simple. But it wouldn't have occurred if I didn't have a partner who was willing to touch me and hold me and attend to me during that time. My tears were just wonderful.

*And, all these people were Hedy and Yumi-ized.*

Hedy- and Yumi-ized. Absolutely. So afterwards they wouldn't leave us. The two women and the technicians came with us everywhere. They just wanted to stick around where we were. They did the chest x-ray, and again let Yumi in there.

*You know, we all feel wonderful in the presence of anyone fully connected to their Core Energy. It makes you want to be around them as much as possible. It feels like home. We resonate to the deliciousness of it. I know it must have felt like a soothing tonic to these technicians who are likely to have had a long list of patients during their shift who are frightened or consumed with pain. Either of those two things automatically keep you from being "connected." Both are at the stick end of the wand. But, along come Hedy and Yumi offering an entirely different vibration at the star end—a vibration of joy and "all is well-ness." No wonder they followed you!*

Well, we had a wonderful, playful time with them.

## *Joy That Went Boom*
### *(Powerful Strategies for Reconnecting)*

The next thing was the bone scan. That is some scary thing! The nuclear medicine department seemed so dismal and un-welcoming.

*Which means, right there, that you have farmed-out some of your Life Force, just focusing on those three things…scary, dismal, and un-welcoming. Those are your cues!*

Uhmm. You know, you're absolutely right.

Once again we were told, "Your husband cannot come in. This is radioactive material," and so on and so on. Well, it turns out that one of the four doctors in nuclear medicine is someone we know very well. In this case, it helped to have a connection, because they agreed to let Yumi in once more. And, you know, we've insisted on this one way or another. In this case I used my connections. In the other case I just went why, why, why, until the rule made no sense. But in this case, I knew I would need to use my connections because they are legally regulated because it's radioactive material.

During the test, we came to another hurdle. When they were finished taking my pictures they called me back in and wanted additional pictures of my pelvis and my shoulder. I thought, "What is all this?" Everything seemed so regimented. The woman doing the test was very cold and official in all her work. Like a robot, working on an inanimate object instead of a human being. When she was done I whispered, "Come close. Tell me why are you taking more pictures." I whispered because I knew I needed to move her a little bit. And she says in a military fashion, "I'm not allowed to say." I said, "Please go back to the doctor and say, 'This patient wants to know why we took more pictures.'" She goes to the doctor and when she returns she says, "The doctor is going to talk to you." It wasn't our friend, it was another one. And he actually showed us the scans. He pointed to the films and showed us where there was a spot on my right shoulder, and a spot on my pelvis. And he said, "It can be trauma, you know, from hitting yourself, falling. It can be degenerative arthritis, or—it can be a tumor." *[In a throaty Groucho Marx manner]:* I said, "Thank you very much!" You know, if you look that close inside of your body you're going to find all kinds of things!

*There, right there is where your energy spiraled downward. I'm willing to bet that if you had gone home before this last test, you would have felt fine. Even though Yumi was allowed to be with you, your attention was first on the bleakness of the nuclear medicine department, then the sergeant-like woman in charge, and finally the questionable test results. All of this amounted to disconnection from your Core Energy. And that means you are out of business. You can't hear spiritual guidance, your energy drops to zero, and you are absolutely overwhelmed. At that moment, if you had been sensitive to how you were feeling and recognized the dip in your well-being, you could have turned it around and sailed through this test just like the others. You could have realized this as merely a disconnection, and that you had the option of pivoting right on the spot. You had the option of thinking better thoughts that would get Life Force flowing once again. It's the sensitivity to how we're feeling that's important. And, the perfect time to ask the perfect question, "What's another way I can look at this?"*

*Better thoughts in response to the noticeable bleakness of the nuclear medicine department, might have been to acknowledge the brilliant minds and extraordinary talent that roam these very halls and operate all this equipment. Like the wonderful doctor who read your mammograms and who spends his time in a dark room looking at films all day. It's probably pretty bleak there, too, and yet it didn't stop you from being aware of his wonderful work. Think of all the miracles that have happened due to the excellent reporting that comes from this very department. Remember that looks are often so deceiving. Perhaps you could look at this bleak department as a diamond in the rough.*

You know, you're right.

*Better thoughts as far as the sergeant-like manner of the woman doing your test might involve pondering what she was like as a toddler. You might notice that she actually takes her work very seriously and is trying to do her very best. You might do the "rocking" technique (the technique mentioned earlier when we were talking about the CAT scan), picturing her as a three-month-old, putting her over your shoulder and rocking her while saying, "All is well," or "Remember who you are." Be ready to notice any signs of softening in her manner. You might engage her in conversation about what she likes best about her work, etc. Whether she changes or not, you must see her differently and feel better about her in order to take back your energy. You can't criticize her and feel wonderful at the same time. We're shooting for "wonderful" here!*

That's for sure!

*When faced with the offsetting test results, you might remember that the body is constantly regaining its balance. It's dynamic. It's programmed for self-healing. And that this test is merely a "freeze-frame" of what they saw at that moment. And that no matter what those spots represent, the very best thing for them in any moment is a continual abundant flow of Life Force, the very thing you pinch off with worry and criticism. You might as well focus on the one possibility the doctor gave you of it being an "old trauma." (Remember the conversation with your waiter on Park Avenue about this diagnosis of cancer being something old that just has to be taken out? This is probably just some "old" injury.) That's the version that will serve you best and get you back in the flow. The flow of well-being is the most important thing you could ever have in any situation. That in itself, is a major healing moment and serves to cover all bases, so to speak! We tend to pick the worst possibility and let it close us down. It's important to throw the process in reverse. Choose the best possibility out of his report and give that your attention. Choose the star end of the magic wand!*

*These are just some ideas for feeling your way back to your center. Just ideas for any future occasions that temporarily throw you off course.*

Those are wonderful examples. Well, needless to say, that night we really had sort of a little bit of a glitch in our path. But once I was rested and thought about it again, I knew that everything was all right.

*Sleep is a perfect way to regain your energy, and to begin again. We automatically re-connect with our Core Energy when we relax and sleep. If we get out of our own way, we sort of "fall into well-being." Sleep is great therapy. It stops that emotional downward spiral, and once again, we have lift-off! When all else fails, take a nap. Even a "napette," (dozing for a few minutes), can help immensely. You might even want to have a wonderful snack when you wake up. Graham crackers and milk are nostalgic for me, just like after our naps in pre-school!*

I truly did feel lighter and stronger after some sleep. And, the next day we called our friend, who is one of the doctors there. He said that he had looked at my films and while they can't say for sure, it is most probably from trauma. If you fall on your coccyx, it'll show as a black area on your x-ray. He said, "I doubt that you have anything to worry about." That was precisely what I needed to hear.

# Chapter 6

# The Boob Dream Team Inductees

That was Friday. We decided that for the Sabbath, we were going to do the first, the second and the fifth commandment all at once. The first commandment is that "I am your God," and we were going to really honor God. The second commandment is "Honor the Sabbath," and we decided that the best way to honor the Sabbath was with Yumi's father. And the fifth commandment is "Honor thy father and thy mother," so we were going to visit him. We drove four-and-a-half hours to Miami and slept on the couch, which was unbelievably uncomfortable, but it was the place we needed to be. We talked to him a little bit and said a few more things. We didn't tell him the whole truth, but he's so smart. He knew something needed to be checked out. We spent the day there, then the next day we drove back very slowly. It was a splendid, splendid day!

The following Monday we drove to Sarasota to visit Robert Walker at the Ellis Cancer Research Center. *[whispering]:* Judie, I mean this is a gorgeous place! Someone donated 17 million dollars to build this wonderful clinic. It's on the top of a hill and the architecture is magnificent. It's not just magnificent, it's actually touching. So much attention was paid to make this a remarkable place. It's not a Taj Mahal. It's just a beautiful, beautiful building.

*A well-spent 17 million.*

Very, very, very well spent. You enter on parquet floors. It seems to be designed with an abundance of natural materials and rounded corners, as if on sort of a human scale. It's just really a very beautiful place. And it doesn't smell like a hospital. It's just clean smelling, which is refreshing. It immediately makes a wonderful impression. As we checked in at the reception desk, the procedure went so smoothly. Everything was extremely well organized. I said to myself, "This is very interesting. There's something going on here." Anyway, we filled out necessary forms and we began waiting, as usual. Once we were called in, for the first time, I wasn't weighed! I said to Yumi, "That's a good sign right there. I may even have a different identity here! Perhaps this time I won't be 'a slightly overweight female'—I will be 'Hedy Schleifer'!"

Then Dr. Walker came into the room. Judie, you **know** when a healer steps in—it's like what we all have the potential to be, but only some of us are. Like you, Robert Walker is a healer. He's this short, somewhat pudgy-in-the-belly, ruddy-complexioned man with reddish-blonde hair, and the warmest eyes...the warmest, deepest, kindest eyes. Well, he came in followed by a resident who sort of stood behind him nervously. And he did doctoring right away. But you know, it was amazing. It fit. It really didn't matter. He had a presence that silently connected his heart with our hearts.

He put up the mammograms, looked at me, and said, "Humh... So you've had a diagnosis that's probably got you in quite a turmoil right now." (See, it was about my mammogram but it was also about me!) He continued, "And you've come here because you're interested in what we're doing, aren't you?" I said, "Oh, I'm incredibly interested. What you're doing is phenomenal." He says, "Well, it is. It is very exciting." And he begins to tell me the story of it: how they came upon it, why they do it, who else is doing it, and what they're doing that's different. He explained that they're trying this way because of recent studies around the country at various centers. One center discovered that the radioactive isotopes will light up the sentinel node and still another one discovered that a blue dye will help guide you. He said, "I've found that if I use the radioactive material to light up the sentinel node so I can pinpoint it, and use the blue dye in the operation, then I just have to make a small incision to get that thing out. And so I'll use both." This combination was the novelty of his approach.

---

## The Human Connection

*He put up the mammograms, and he looked at me and said, "Humh... So you've had a diagnosis that's probably got you in quite a turmoil right now."*

*(See, it was about my mammogram, but it was also about me!)*

---

Anyway, he settled into his chair and told us the whole story. His hands were on top of my chart and films of my mammogram, and he just kept his eyes focused on us as he spoke.

And I said, "You have a vision, don't you? And you're really going after it." And he said, "Yes, I do." He was all puffed up, obviously filled with delight and actually blushed. He just got all red. I just loved him.

*Ahh, do I detect that you have sniffed out a member of your Boob Dream Team?*

Absolutely. I said, "You know, you are one who knows breast mapping, and I am the one who knows mensch mapping. You know, a mensch in Yiddish is a 'full human being.' A mensch is the highest thing you can say about a person. You, Robert Walker, are definitely a mensch!" And he blushed again.

Meanwhile, the resident relaxes. *[whispering]:* I said to the resident, "This is some doctor." He said, "I know. I've been watching him in awe." I said, "I understand. He is a <u>real</u> doctor."

Anyway, an hour later, he had finished explaining everything. He says, "So, Hedy, what do you think? Do you want to do this? Do you want to have a lumpectomy?" Then he explained, "A lumpectomy will remove the lesion and then we'll take out the one node." He says, "The one thing about your case is that, out of 261 women, we've only had 14 who had a medial lesion (located on the side of the breast nearer the sternum or breast bone). Usually the lesions are on the outer portion. What we don't know yet is how many of those drain to a sentinel node under the rib cage which holds the mammary sentinel node, and how many of them drain into the axillary sentinel node. We just don't know. And if they drain to the mammary sentinel node, we can't get it because it's underneath the rib cage and we have to use a different strategy. In our studies, we've found that this has been a hidden place of metastasis. That's why, with some people who have had a mastectomy, the malignancy would return again. It was in that sentinel node underneath the rib cage."

He says something like, "With you, given that the lesion is on the medial side, I don't know. Is it going to go here? Is it going to go there? If it's in the mammary sentinel node, we have a more complicated situation. If it isn't, it's pretty simple."

Well, you know, it's nice to be talked to like that, you know what I'm saying? It's like you're a partner and—I said, "What are the chances of it going here?" He says, "Fifty-fifty. You are the fourteenth woman. We've had seven in the axillary sentinel node (under the arm), and six in the mammary sentinel node (underneath the rib cage)."

I said, "Well, let's take a chance."

Then, to our surprise and delight, a wonderful friend of ours popped in, who also turned out to be on the staff at Ellis. He had been in our couples' workshops. He said to Dr. Walker, "Robert, these people are phenomenal. They saved my marriage. I've gone to their seminar twice. They're family. I adore them." This was really delicious. Here was Robert Walker, a devout Mormon, and our other friend, who is a Jew. And the devout Mormon is short and stocky and the Jew is long and tall, and they are so funny together. And they are partners in this, partners who quickly became my Boob Dream Team. And they really are the Boob Dream Team. This just got better and better!

Our friend then took us to the radiation oncologist. We talked to him and I quickly realized that **this** is what I was looking for. He took a piece of paper and said, "I'm going to write these things down so you will be sure to have it; otherwise you might not remember it because you are too excited. And it's going to be about you, Hedy." He just wrote down everything that had to do with the breast and what radiation would mean, and then he said, "I'm making your post-operative report out right now. It says that it's my guess that your sentinel node is clear." Good. How many doctors would take a chance on making such a bold statement? How many people would take a chance like this outside of a university setting? You know, most would be afraid of legal repercussions. He said, "My sense is that the margins are clear." At the end of the report he says, "Hedy, you've got a good report card here!" So that was like, "All right!"

*Cells smiling!*

Absolutely. My whole body loved hearing this proposed report about Hedy! You know, this is real medicine. His best sense said that I would be fine. This would be my report; he knew it. He looked at me. He could see!

## A Mother's Gift

So, yesterday our friend Ted called again and left a lovely message. I returned his call today and I said, "Ted, let me tell you what has happened." *[softly]:* I said, "You know, in all of this we have gone with our inspiration. From the very beginning, we began to notice that there was a stone placed in front of every footstep, and we just put our foot on one stone, followed by another. It wasn't like we had to do something. There it was, and we put our foot on it. And we have found the most amazing team," I said. "It's the Boob Dream Team—**the Boob Dream Team!**" *[Judie, roaring with laughter]* And I told him a brief version of our recent journey in which we found just the perfect team through our inspiration.

*[whispering]:* He said, "Hedy, you are like your mother. *[Hedy's mother is a visionary, a remarkable woman who survived the holocaust...one miracle at a time.]* I have tears," he said, as he began to cry. He went on, "Hedy, you are just like your mother. You can step into something, and you grab it with your whole being—the grace, the inspiration, the elegance, and the faith with which you, you and Yumi, have just taken this thing on." He said, "I can't help but wonder, what kind of a mother your mother had, to have nurtured these qualities in her—and what kind of mother you have that passed on such priceless gifts." And he was just crying.

And I said, "Ted, you're right. It is my mother. I hadn't thought about, you know, stepping into this event. I was just doing what I saw her do, and what I know she did during the war and during those dark years, where she just stepped in and created Light wherever she was...which at that time was right in the middle of the German Prison Camp. She was able to create miracles right in the midst of unspeakable drama. You know, the uniforms meant nothing to her. She knew that there was a human being inside and she connected with the human being. Like my mother, I see that there is not only a doctor in this lab coat, there is a human being in there. I must speak to the human being."

*Yeah!*

You know, the white coat, the uniform, who **cares about that**!

*Absolutely!*

## A Mother's Gift

*My mother stepped in and created Light wherever she was... which at one time, was right in the middle of the German Prison Camp.*

*She was able to create miracles, right in the midst of unspeakable drama. You know, the uniforms meant nothing to her. She knew that there was a human being inside, and she connected with the human being.*

*Like my mother, I see that there is not only a doctor in this lab coat, there's a human being in there! I must speak to the human being.*

*You know Hedy, as you paraded around, searching for the Boob Dream Team, looking past the white coat, you stimulated such a rich exchange. You regained your power by seeing past the uniform and into the human being, who really wanted to help you in the best way they knew how. They in turn, were in all likelihood, moved to think and speak from a freshly inspired place deep inside them. People love that feeling of reconnection as they shift into who they really are, and more accurately match the vision of who they hoped they'd be as human beings—as humans being physicians—before the protocol and overly-booked schedules were added. If you had just been "saying" empty words, it wouldn't have moved anyone. You were "being it." You and Yumi appeared before them fully connected to who you are. You initially watched to see which people "showed up" in your life, and it simultaneously led you to show up unexpectedly in the lives of others. In just moments, there were enormous, mutual benefits for each of you; not to mention benefits for the patients following you, who will possibly receive a higher level of inspired human presence within their medical experience. As for the rare instance when the experience was less than what you'd prefer, you moved right on, never looking back. You didn't even reference them again* in casual conversation. "Carrying on" about imperfection in others holds you back, and robs you of your energy. It's like that vision of running full-throttle towards the Light (all you consider sacred), while sporting a long trail of toilet paper stuck to your foot! You, Hedy, made a clean leap with each visit and went right on to the next possibility. You searched, resonated, made an inspired connection, and RELEASED what didn't serve you. A wonderfully clean leap. Now <u>THAT'S</u> living!

Yes. Yes! [laughing]

---

### Those Who Didn't Make the Boob Dream Team

"Carrying on" about imperfection in others only holds you back and robs you of your energy. It's like the vision of running full-throttle towards the Light (all you consider sacred and wonderful), while sporting a long trail of toilet paper stuck to your foot!

You, Hedy, made a clean leap with each visit and went right on to the next possibility. You searched, resonated, made inspired connections, and RELEASED what didn't serve you. A wonderfully clean leap! Now THAT'S living!

# Chapter 7

# Encountering the Sacred Right Where You Are

So they set up the surgery. The woman who sets it up is an angel. I mean, I'm telling you these angel stories, but this woman is *[drawn out in song]*: a—vail—able! She was like an attentive mommy. She said, "Come sit in my office, and we'll set you up for Wednesday."

We went from there to the surgery admissions desk and gave them the necessary information. The woman who was there was just a riot. She was just the funniest person. She says, "Hedy, from 12 midnight until 8 a.m., only clear liquids: Jell-O, tea or black coffee, clear juice, etc." Yumi says, "Is semen a clear liquid?" She was immediately on the floor with laughter. She just couldn't believe that he had said that. Well, Dr. Walker came over. She says, "Dr. Walker, after instructing clear liquids for the day of surgery, I was just asked by this gentleman whether semen is a clear liquid?" And he blushed again and laughed. She was having so much fun with this story. She spread the story around. We could tell here and there that the word was out and that others were quietly saying, "That's the couple with the oral sex, you know, with the clear liquids." There was an atmosphere of such joy and comfort, and I think it's Robert Walker's doing. I think that whole department has his imprimatur. Everybody is relaxed and makes real contact.

So that was Monday. That was also when I told you that I was going to go to sleep that night with four beautiful angels surrounding me. You know, you laugh about your three angels: Flo, Clarity and Inspiration, the girls, as you call them. And I have four others: Michael, Raphael, Uriel, and Gabriel. My four angels surrounded me that night. When I awakened, I was inspired. I knew this plan was right. I knew I was on the right track.

That day, we went to Clearwater Beach, getting the last room available at the hotel. It's a gorgeous old hotel from the twenties. We saw a breath-taking sunset that evening, followed by a stunning sunrise the next morning. It was incredible. We made love and just had a beautiful time. It was just the perfect preparation to ready us for the next day.

And then I read your stuff you had faxed to me. It truly inspired me, Judie, to ask myself, "How do I want to spend this morning, the day of my surgery? How would I orchestrate this day?" After the sunrise, I took a walk, had a wonderful bath and began planning. What do I want to do? And I laid out my day.

---

## *Sacred Intentions (Designing a Fabulous Day!)*

*And I thought, "How do I want to spend this morning, the day of my surgery?"*
*...After the sunrise, a walk, and a wonderful bath...*
*What do I want to do? I laid out my day.*

---

Let's see. I want to call Alice MacMahon and thank her for creating the wonderful Florida Hospital Women's Center; because of her and this wonderful center, this was early detection. So I want to call her. I want to call our friend who had the heart problem, and let him know I'm going into surgery and afterwards his heart better be beating beautifully! I want to fax a letter to another friend who's going into surgery for his liver and lungs and include your letter. I want to talk to the friend of ours in New York who gave us the doctor that helped us turn the corner. I made the list and I just went down the list. Everybody was home, almost as if they were waiting for my call. It all seemed pre-orchestrated. I mean, it was like charmed. I did all of that, that morning.

Yumi was driving, and the car just "drove itself," all the way to Ellis. Yumi even noticed it. We arrived effortlessly. The admissions process was unbelievable. This Spanish woman with this broad smile greeted us warmly. I said to her, "You know, you are the perfect person to have in admittance for a thing like this. You are bright and cheery and lively and sociable." And she says, "Well, thank you. I'm just doing my job." I said, "Ah, ah, ah, ah. It could be done a lot of different ways." The whole procedure is all designed so well. She took care of us in a separate little area with lots of privacy. She had pictures surrounding her of her beautiful little grandchildren. The admissions procedure went so smoothly.

## "We Saw a Little Star Twinkling in my Axilla!"

Then it was on to nuclear medicine for the first procedure. This is where the lesion would be injected with radioactive isotopes. It had to be done three hours before the operation. Suddenly, this guy shows up. Immediately, I noticed that he didn't seem to fit here. It was like he must have been from another hospital.

He said (sergeant-like), "Schleifer?"

I said, "Yes."

He said, "Please come back."

And I said, "Can my husband come?" "No." (Here we go again! By now, I knew Yumi could go in.)

I said, "Why not?"

"Florida law."

I said, "Why?" "Radioactive material."

"Oh, so there's no way of breaking that rule?"

"Of course not." "Okay." So I left it. I knew this was not the end.

So I was put into a little room on this little gurney and I'm waiting, and I remembered what you said in your paper about "filling your mind with wonderful thoughts." That morning, another call I made was to Yumi's aunt, our favorite aunt in New York. She's marvelous. And she says, "Hedy, I'm going to read the Psalms on the subway as I go to work." It's called a Tehilim in Hebrew. She's an Orthodox Jew with this funny wig, and I could just see her on the subway reading the Psalms. I could see her. So I'm thinking, "Judie said think of wonderful things." So I just kept picturing my aunt, her wig, and her reading the Psalms. I was sitting there grinning from ear to ear from the vision. Instead of feeling absolutely alone and afraid, I just filled my mind with this beautiful picture. I told her later how that was such a fantastic gift.

Then this young woman, Sharon, comes in and I'm grinning from ear to ear. She says, "What's with you?"

I said, "Well, I'm just thinking about my aunt, you know, who is saying the Psalms today while riding on the subway."

And she's still sort of a little proper, and she says, "Has Dr. Walker explained this procedure to you?"

I said, "Explained it to me?" I said, "Absolutely. Sharon, I am so excited to be here. Not only has he explained it to me but this research means so much to me."

She says, "It does? It means a lot to me, too." And she begins to carry on a conversation. Eventually I said, "Sharon, can you break the rule? Can you break the law and bring my husband in?" She says, "Is this going to mean a lot to you?"

I said, "Sharon, it's going to mean the world to me! As a matter of fact, it means everything to me!"

She says, "Let me go talk to the doctor." She comes back and says, "He can come in."

So, of course, he came right in, and we talked while she was setting everything up. Then the doctor arrived. Judie, listen to this. She's a woman of substance, and gray hair in the amount of which I have never seen in my life, pulled back in a big French braid. I took one look at her and I said, "You are the doctor who said my husband could come in, aren't you?" She smiled and said, "I'll do anything I can that will make a patient even 10 percent more comfortable." She said, "I break every rule." I said, "You are fantastic." I said, "What about this gray hair of yours? Isn't this something!" And we're having this immediate, personal conversation. "I can't believe you are old enough to have gray hair!" And she said, "I'm young, but my hair fools a lot of people."

## *Let's Break the Rules!*

*I took one look at her and I said,*
*"You are the doctor who said my husband could*
*come in, aren't you?" She smiled and said,*
*"I'll do anything I can that will make*
*a patient even 10 percent more comfortable."*
*She says, "I break every rule."*

Then I said, "Listen, I'm unbelievably excited about what you are all doing with this research, and I just feel so honored to be part of it." And so she explained some more about it. Then she showed the technician (who couldn't feel the lump when she tried earlier) how to feel for this tiny lump. Like all the doctors there, she is a professor and they teach constantly. It was truly beautiful to watch.

Then she injected the radioactive isotopes. We watched in awe as it showed up on the screen, steadily outlining absolute magnificence in human design. Our bodies are so fabulous. Yumi and I watched silently, and breathlessly, as magical radioactive isotopes traveled right to the node. *[high-pitched and in delight]*: And there it was, that little node. It was like a star, twinkling! I mean, we had tears in our eyes. *[drawn out and emphatically]*: The way the <u>body</u> is de-<u>signed</u> with that little twinkling sentinel, that's actually watching over that part of you. I said, "That's incredible. This is the most amazing thing I've ever seen." We were just in awe.

*Don't you even like the name? Every time you even say the name, "Sen-ti-nel node," it sounds so regal!*

## A Little Star Twinkling in my Axilla!

*Yumi and I watched silently, and breathlessly,
as magical radioactive isotopes traveled
right to the node. [high pitched and in delight]:
And there it was. There was that little node.
It was like a star, twinkling!
I mean we had tears in our eyes.
[drawn out and emphatically]:
The way the <u>body</u> is de-<u>signed</u>
with that little twinkling sentinel,
that's actually watching over that part of you.*

Yes. It's so special. And, of course, to have Yumi and me so excited about the magic and wisdom of the human body and the magic and wisdom of this research. It was obvious that they were thrilled, and so were we.

## The Divine Shake-Down!

Everything that followed had that kind of magic, Judie. It's like you were saying…it seems like the more you appreciate, the more wonderful stuff is delivered to you. When the test was complete, they wheeled me into a surgical area and they brought warm blankets! It was so comforting. All these warm blankets snuggling up against me.

*You know, that's a wonderful memory of mine, as well, from a minor surgery I had years ago. Such a small but profound gesture! A warm "all is well" blanket!*

That's just how I felt...so well-cared for. Oh, that feeling. All is well. And the pace. From the time I arrived there, Judie, the pace was so perfect that I could integrate every part of what was being done. When she started the intravenous, she did it in slow, informative steps. Slow—now, this is what we're giving you and this is why. And when the nurse brought the blankets, she gently opened the curtain. She said, *[playfully faking a French accent]:* "Ma-dam. I brought your warm blankets!" This funny, playful woman. And so they asked me how much sedation I wanted and I said, "The least possible. I really want to be awake." And they said, "Fine."

*You wanted to be a participant.*

Completely, in everything. They did the lumpectomy, and when they were done they looked down and said, "Hedy, the node is clear." And I just began to cry. I just cried, and I thanked them. I said, "Thank you. Thank you. Thank you!"

As they wheeled me out, I began to shake and cry at the same time. And the nurse said, "Would you like some medication?" And I said, "Oh no! This is the best thing. I want to shake and cry for as long as I need to shake and cry!" And she said, "Do you need anything?" And I said, "Well, I do. Could you come close and hold my hand?" And she said, "Of course. Of course." So she held my hand. Then she had something to do and she came back and she held my hand. And I just kept shaking. My whole body shook. I was also still crying. I looked up at this wonderful nurse who was holding my hand and said, "This is just release. This is a release of fear and tension and at the same moment profound gratefulness and happiness. This is just a release. Just hold my hand." When I was done with that, I was so peaceful. Noticing this she said, "You know, you've just taught me something so important. We've been medicating patients when they began shaking, not realizing that all they might need is to have their hand held." I said to her, "My whole body is just so relaxed. My mind is relaxed. My heart is relaxed. You've just helped me discharge all of that stuff." And she said, "Thank you. This has been such an important lesson for me." So I said, "You know, some people may prefer to be medicated. That's a different story. But, now that you know about this, you can give them other options and let them know how natural that is. They may have a very different feeling about what they would choose."

## The Divine Shake-Down!

*As they wheeled me out, I began to shake and cry at the same time. And the nurse said, "Would you like some medication?"*

*And I said, "Oh no! This is the best thing. I want to shake and cry for as long as I need to shake and cry!"*

*And she said, "Do you need anything?" And I said, "Well, I do. Could you come close and hold my hand?"*

Then they took me to the room where Yumi was waiting for me, and I felt marvelous. It was late in the afternoon. In nearly every area, our whole experience seemed to be orchestrated to perfection. There were perhaps two people, out of twenty-two, who weren't team players. They were off playing solitaire! They were the young man in the radiology department who bellowed stubbornly, "That's the law," and a doctor the next morning, who suddenly threw open the blinds, robotically looked at my incision, wrote an order that I could be discharged, and left. But everyone else came in, looked into my eyes and warmly said things like, "How are you doing?" Often they touched me gently at the same time. These were the star players on my Boob Dream Team!

*[whispering]*: And then, after that, we went to a condo at the beach and had this very special recovery there. It was perfect. You know, just walking around bare-breasted and letting in the air and the sun...and feeling the beauty and strength of the ocean.

## Two Hearts, One Voice... and a Life-Changing Visit

Yesterday we went for the postoperative visit. We entered the waiting room.

*Appropriately named—I've often pondered who might hold the record for the longest wait! There should be some sort of a score board, perhaps with pictures and initials of the winners!*

*[laughing]* Yes, you wait, and you wait! We waited for an hour-and-a-half. But, Yumi and I really know how to wait. I had taken a large bag that contained all the cards and letters I had received. Prior to this, there had been no time (or I hadn't made time) to read them. Some were sympathy cards and said sad things. It's like...who wants to read THAT! Some of them were thoughts, you know, like "We're with you," and "We know your power and

---

### What's in a Name?
#### (Perfection!...and an Open Valve!)

*I want to make contact with this woman.
"What happened to you?" I asked.
"They took out my whole larynx...I think I'm doing
fantastic largely because I have
a wonderful monthly support group
called The Chatter Boxes!"*

your strength to overcome anything." You know. Suddenly, I opened up this card that had lots of tiny purple hearts loose in it.

Shortly after we had arrived, I noticed a woman sitting two chairs down from us. She had a small device that she used in order to speak; her voice came out sounding like a machine. And when I got this bunch of hearts I thought, "I want to make contact with this woman." So I said, "Would you like a purple heart?" "Oh," she says, "Yes, I would love a purple heart!" (You know, with her machine.) Then she took it.

And then I read a printout of a joke someone had e-mailed to me. It was the funniest thing. I said to this woman, "Would you like to have a belly laugh?" and I gave it to her. She loved the joke.

We began to have a conversation and I said, "What did they do to you?" And she says, "Well, they took out my whole larynx [voice box]," this, that, and the other.

And I said, "How are you doing?"

And she says, "Fantastic. I think I'm doing fantastic because of my wonderful support group." (All of this is said while using her little machine.) "And," she says, "We have a support group that meets once a month. Everyone in the group has had their larynx removed. We call our group The Chatter Boxes!"

I said, "That's phenomenal."

Anyway, she says it has helped her tremendously. And then she told me the most amazing story. She said that when they were wheeling her off to surgery, her husband was at her side. He said, "Would you tell me one more time that you love me? Because this is the last time I'm going to hear your voice this way."

And she continued, "So I said, **I love you, I love you, I love you!**" And she's saying this with the machine.

And she says, "I screamed it over and over as they wheeled me into the operating room so it would be branded in his mind."

To think that I would never have met this woman had I not been on this journey! Never! In all the years of my life, I would not have met her. And she said to me, "Hedy, I'm going to put this little purple heart in my purse, in my change purse, and I will keep it forever. Since I've had to use this device to speak, people don't approach me to have conversations. I have to approach them. And you just approached me, and gave me this purple heart, and we had this big conversation and," she said, "I'll never forget this." What a moment!

## The Priceless Gift of Precious Words...

*(While this woman is on her way into surgery for a laryngectomy, her husband asks:)*

*"Because this is the last time I'm going to hear your voice, would you tell me one more time that you love me?" So I said,*
**"I love you, I love you, I love you!"**
*as they wheeled me into the operating room. I screamed it so it would be branded in his mind.*

# Chapter 8

# Decisions, Decisions... Inspired Decisions!

*[A few weeks later, we meet once more in my kitchen to talk.]*

*[slowly and warmly]:* Once again, I want to call the angels of healing, the angels of clarity, flow, and inspiration and ask that we be guided to speak beautiful words of wisdom—treasured thoughts and reflections that will touch the lives of others and massage them into their wholeness. For that is the gift; we honor that and say thank you. Hedy, what would you like to add?

*[softly]:* M-m-m-m. Just thank you. This is so wonderful. Amen!

*Amen. Here we are, talking to the spatula again!*

It's just perfect! Well, since I saw you last time, the "news" is very interesting. As you know, I have been healing phenomenally from this operation, the lumpectomy, the taking out of the cyst, and the three nodes that they cut out. The healing is phenomenal. I will show it to you. You will be pret–ty a–mazed! The scars are nearly invisible. My breast looks fantastic, and I feel great. Every once in a while, if we drive over a bump I can feel a little tenderness inside my breast, but it really is healing fantastically. And I know it really is because I had the perfect combination of feeling in charge and surrendering to treatment. And that combination, that paradox, of feeling the two emotions simultaneously is phenomenal! *[picking up speed dramatically]:* Feeling **completely in control and in charge** and surrendering... it is really a phenomenal thing. And everything in me is just healing beautifully.

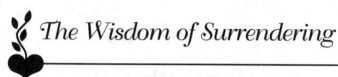

### *The Wisdom of Surrendering*

*My breast is really healing fantastically,*
*and I know it really is because*
*I had the perfect combination of*
***feeling in charge***
***and surrendering***
*to treatment.*

I was on top of the world, even a little bit cocky, I think. I was just sort of the "bitch on wheels" about this thing, you know. *[laughing]* And, in looking back on some of the conversations I had, I'm a bit embarrassed because I was sort of brazen, and aach! You know... Well, two things happened at once.

The doctor called, not my surgeon but his assistant, and the laboratory results arrived by way of our office fax machine. I have new advice! Even though Yumi and I like to participate as fully as possible in medical decisions, you should think twice before reading a doctor's laboratory reports without an explanation. It can look very bad on paper. This looked very bad. It actually looked like the sentinel node had metastasized and that it measured .9 centimeters, which is pretty big. And it didn't even occur to us logically, at that point, that if it had been that large, they would have seen it right away. But you know, you aren't thinking logically. We just panicked. We absolutely panicked.

And the doctor said, "You have to come right away, and as soon as you get here, beep me."

### *Frightening Facts—Faxed!*

*I have new advice:
People should think twice before reading
a doctor's laboratory reports
without an explanation because
it can look very bad on paper.
This looked very bad.*

I also happen to have an office manager who is easily undone when something bad happens, and you know, she just got very scared about it. In this case, now three of us were panicking. Yumi and I immediately left for Sarasota. We were trying to wave our imaginary magic wand, trying hard to stay at the star end. We waved it with momentary success, thinking better thoughts, and then it would suddenly flip on us, and we'd spiral downward with our "what if's." Then we'd notice that we were at the stick end again and we'd start fresh. At least we knew what to strive for, and had that to guide us. I think we did phenomenally well, considering.

I called my son who lives in New York and we talked a little bit. I said, "I don't know what this is all about, but this is what we know so far. We'll call when we find out more." And he said, "Mom, it's just time to mobilize again." *[whispering]:* He's so wonderful.

*Perfect. Perfect!*

It's just time to mobilize again! I also talked to a cousin in New York who is wonderful. But, that's all. I decided not to tell the whole world because I didn't even know the whole story. And I didn't want to give this unpleasant possibility more energy, especially MY energy. I knew we had to stay as connected as possible.

After a drive that seemed to take forever, we finally arrived. It turned out that this time we would be seen by a young resident. We told him that we had seen the report and he said, "Oh, okay. I don't know how you got it, because I just found out. But, here is what's going on." And he drew on a piece of paper. He said that this is a microscopic trace of cancer. It is so small that two out of three people didn't see it. But it is in one nodule of a node." Actually, it was a tiny speck on one of the many nodules of one node. Because this university researches microscopic cancer, they found it. He says, "And so, you're going to need surgery. You're going to have to have all your nodes removed." And I looked at Yumi and it was like, *[in a soft whimper]:* oh! no! I don't want surgery. I don't want more surgery! And something in my body said, "No, we're not doing that." But that was a reaction, it wasn't an inspiration. It was a reaction. It was like, I'm not having more surgery! It was resistance. Anyway, we decided to schedule it only because you can always cancel. So, it was scheduled, and I received all the necessary instructions for the surgery.

## *The Decision...and the "Aha!"*
## *(regarding further surgery)*

Then we went to the other doctor, the radiation oncologist. The team over there is extraordinary. The doctor said warmly, "Come into my office." It was as if no one else existed. He began to explain the whole situation. Soon it became clear to Yumi on a scientific level, and clear to me on a spiritual level, that I didn't need this operation. What's interesting is that we came to this same conclusion simultaneously. The data he presented was kind of above my head, but Yumi with his scientific mind, easily understood it. Yumi was listening very carefully. Just as I was saying "I don't feel I need this operation," slowly but surely,

## *Reaction...Not Inspiration*

*And I looked at Yumi...it was like,*
*(in a soft whimper) "Oh! No! I don't want surgery!"*
*And something in my body said,*
*"No, we're not doing that!"*
*But, that was a reaction...*
*it wasn't inspiration.*

Yumi said, "Given this, this, and this and this, it seems to me that Hedy doesn't need this operation." But, for me, it was inspiration from within, and for him it was pure logic.

And the doctor said, "Well, that is certainly a decision she could make." He couldn't openly support this choice because this is a research hospital and, you know, they really want the data on microscopic cancer. They want that data. He continued hesitatingly, "Well...yes, that certainly..." And Yumi and I looked at each other like, "Aha! There isn't going to be an operation!"

Anyway, the Kosher Choreographer lined everything up perfectly once again. During this visit, our friend who's an oncologist there, popped in. He sat with us during the meeting and held my hand. As we were having these insights, he squeezed my hand. And I thought, "He knows something." Soon after that, he had to leave. Later, as Yumi and I were leaving the office, suddenly, there he was again. He was going to be interviewed on television shortly, but he said, "Come with me in the elevator." And I said, "Yumi and I, as you saw, came to the conclusion that we don't need..." And he interrupted, saying, "Let's talk tonight." But he's smiling. He didn't want to say too much. There were a lot of people around.

We came home and I called our son and I said, "Yigal, they said I have to have an operation. I'm not having an operation. My body is telling me I don't need this operation."

## *Levels of Clarity... Leading to Connection*

*It became clear to Yumi
on a scientific level, and
to me on a Spiritual level, that
I didn't need this operation.*

He said, "Oh, Mom. Are you sure? It's scary when doctors say you need to have an operation and it's cancer."

I said, "Yep. I am. I'm sure. I am going to ask other people, but I'm sure." I said, "I'm still going to talk to a few more people, because I just want to see what's out there. From inside I know already. But let me see what's out there."

That night we called our friend, who was the dean of the medical school, and told him about it all. He got very upset. In a loud, sergeant-like tone he said, "Have you talked to your surgeon about that? You have to talk to your surgeon. And I will check into that. *[even louder]:* You know, the fact that you're afraid of an operation doesn't mean you shouldn't have it."

I said softly, "It's not out of fear. It's out of inspiration." But, I don't think he could hear what I was saying.

Later that night, we got to talk to our friend, the oncologist. And he said with a lilt in his voice, "Hedy, you're right. You don't need this operation. They will want you to have this operation. They really do need the data, but you, in your specific case, do not need this operation."

I said, "Oh, thank you."

But, I was still sort of curious, you know, about what other people out there know. So we went back to our woman doctor friend in Vero Beach on the way to visit Yumi's father again that weekend. And, you'll recall, she's the one who turned us on to the sentinel node. So Yumi said, "Let's go see her. She seems to be a very bright light for us." After a thorough explanation of recent events, we said, "What do you think?" She said, "Hedy, you don't need this operation. You don't. I would recommend chemotherapy because you still have your menstrual period, and your body is producing so much estrogen and so much progesterone which feed cells that grow fast and, you know, you're so hormonal." She's right. I am. I'm high on progesterone. I'm high on estrogen. I'm high on testosterone. I'm high on ev-ery-thing! And my body is in a feeding frenzy. And she said, "You're better off to have chemotherapy, just as an insurance. You may be cured right now. It's just that we don't know for sure, and this is insurance." "Ah," I said, "Thanks to you I will have a wonderful weekend. Yumi and I have made a decision. This weekend we'll put cancer out the window. We're not talking about it. We're just going to have a wonderful weekend with his father. And on Monday we'll study; we'll 'go back to school' and study chemo."

So we did just that. Every time it came knocking at the door we said, "Oh, hi," *[laughing]* and then we sent it on out the window. We just let it go.

*That was so wise.*

---

### Cancer Goes Out the Window! (Hello...goodbye!)

*"This weekend we'll put cancer out the window.*
*We're just going to have a*
*wonderful weekend with Yumi's father.*
*And on Monday we'll go*
*'back to school' and study chemo."*
*So we did just that. But every time it came*
*knocking at the door, we said, "Oh, hi," [laughing]*
*and then we sent it on out the window.*

---

You know, we didn't discuss it. There was nothing to discuss. We knew we had made the right decision. It was clear.

# *Searching for the Perfect Cocktail...Party!*

I had another appointment with an oncologist in Orlando, an oncologist who has helped my friend Linda come back from near death after a diagnosis of cancer. She was dying. Truly.

*The one who went down to 90 pounds and was in a coma?*

The very one! I spent one day each week with her. I crawled up into bed with her and just held her against me and loved her. Another friend and I were just consistently with her—we touched her and loved her and kissed her. I mean, she didn't recognize any of us anymore. And you know, with the combination of everything...she's come back!

*It's as if you loved her into wholeness, or into wellness!*

Precisely. Her doctor also sent her to a university hospital, and they did something there. And I don't know if it's that, or what we did, or the combination. But she's back and doing fabulous. Now she's getting her body back. Her hearing is coming back. She has hair once again and has dyed it a new color. Unbelievable! We worked hard with her.

*That's just so fabulous!*

## *Hedy's Gift to Linda*

*(Linda was terminally ill,
down to 90 pounds and in a coma.)*

*I spent a day each week with her.
I crawled up into bed with her and
just held her against me and loved her.
Now, she's come back and is doing fabulous! It's like
loving her into wholeness, or loving her into wellness!*

So I went to see Linda's doctor. And as I entered his waiting room, I was suddenly overwhelmed. It was filled to capacity with people who were obviously dealing with cancer. What a place! My whole body closed up. Then we waited, you know, in that room. And, as I've said before, Yumi and I know how to wait. We know how to make contact with people, and we talk to little children, and all that. But still, it was a very unpleasant room, and it was one of those doctors' offices where there's a glass cage for the office staff. They open up the window and they close it. They stick out a little piece of paper and they close it.

Anyway, we met this doctor. A nice man, just a very nice man. But harried, so harried. I mean, you can see that he's got 90 people all over on chemo, on this and on that, and he's really stretched in all directions. And so Yumi and I took some time and we just paused and looked at him, you know. And we took some deep breaths, and he relaxed. And he said, "So you're Linda's friend." And I said, "Yes." He said, "I wish I could have more turn out like she did. What a nice turn-around!"

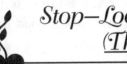

## *Stop—Look—and Breathe!* *(Then begin!)*

*So I went to see Linda's doctor.*
*And as I entered his waiting room, I was suddenly overwhelmed. It was filled to capacity with people who were obviously dealing with cancer. What a place!*
*My whole body closed up.*
*(There's your "Cue!" Your valve is closed.)*

And then he explained everything about chemo, and it was a very good lecture. He really explained it to us, and took all the time in the world. And then he said it would be every three weeks, and this is the regimen, and this is the reason, etc.

And Yumi says, "Well, could we travel?"

"Oh, no, you cannot travel, because, you know, you need to be close and, you know, I can't take any chances, and—"

Yumi said, "Okay." You know, it looked like, if we chose him, we'd be stuck here for the next four months. And I said, "And where does the chemotherapy take place?" He showed us the area where chemotherapy is given.

*[lowering her voice and slowing her words]:* Judie, his office is like a maze.

And in part of the maze, is this room without windows,
  there are eight synthetic leather armchairs,
   a television is blaring,
    people are sitting,
     and nurses going back and forth doing other stuff.

*[softly and confidentially]:* I took one look and I thought, "Unh-uh, unh-uh, unh-uh."

He says, "Oh, you know, at our other location we have windows." I said, "Oh, that's good." Anyway, we left. I said to Yumi, "This is a nice man. He is a good doctor. I know he's a good doctor. But this is not the place—"

*Not the place for you!*

Not for me! But what a gift it provided in clarifying what I wanted by way of seeing what I didn't want. You know, one of those backward gifts in disguise.

## *Expansion of the Boob Dream Team!*

Anyway, then we drove to Sarasota, and I don't know, that place is just sacred to me. That place is **sa-cred**! We arrived there. First of all, they're our friends, and we are their friends. They're thrilled to see us, we're thrilled to see them.

First of all, I met a new physician—a young, wonderful woman with radiant eyes, wonderful face, wonderful touch. She said, "You don't need to get undressed. Stay dressed, we need to talk."

*Ohhh . . . Woah!*

We sat around a table. We just talked. And the first thing she said was, "You know, if you decide on chemo, and that is really your decision, Hedy, I'll tell you all about it today, but it is your decision." (Ahhh, so lovely!) She said, "First, I want to tell you all the things we have to really counteract possible side effects. For nausea we have this, and for this we have that, and we can make you really comfortable. And my intent is, whatever you choose, I am here to make you comfortable. Chemotherapy is a big commitment. It has a price, and I want you to be completely comfortable." And then she laid out everything and took her time.

She's got this phenomenal nurse. And the two of them are like the odd couple. She's very peaceful and quiet, and the nurse is hyperactive and full of fun. *[sounding like a tape playing on fast-forward as she mimics the nurse]:* The nurse is there saying, "Okay, are you still talking to these people?" "Yeah." "Okay, there's more people waiting, but they can wait because you need to talk to these people, but I'll let them know that you want to talk to people!" And she was saying all this in front of us—she's very funny and just marvelous. And I'm thinking, "Umm, I'm in the right place."

*Absolutely.*

Anyway, we talked and talked and talked, and as we were talking, I could feel how right this was for me. This is important insurance. Chemotherapy is important insurance. This is what they know how to do in '97. In the year 2000, they'll do something else, but in '97 they don't know how to give people any other kind of insurance, other than this one.

## *Expanding the Boob Dream Team!*

*I met a new physician for my team,*
*a young, wonderful woman*
*with radiant eyes, wonderful face, wonderful touch.*
*She began,*
*"No, you don't need to get undressed.*
*Stay dressed, we need to talk."*
*We sat around a table. We just talked.*
*And I'm thinking,*
*"I'm in the right place!"*

And then Yumi said, "Can we travel?" And she said, "But of course you can travel. If you go to Israel, I'll make sure I make contact with a doctor over there." She says, "I don't know about the jet lag. You know, Hedy will need to take good care of herself, but if that's exactly what the two of you want to do, I'll be in touch with them and I'll fax them and I'll be..." And Yumi and I look at each other, reflecting on the difference between this and a harried doctor who is saying, *[loud and bold]:* "Don't bother me with your travels and don't bother me with your unique situation. I have enough with my 90 people." You know, with her it's like ev-ery-body is an in-di-vid-ual. And I thought, "Wow." I'm not going to travel, but it's nice to know that she will do anything.

And then she said, "Well, the place for the chemo is across the street." It's late. (They stayed 'til 7:00 p.m. for us.) And Yumi said, "What does it look like?" And she said, "Well, it's a big room, and there are chairs sort of positioned in such a way that people can have their privacy." Yumi said, "Do you have private rooms?" She said, "You know, if you two want a private room, we'll arrange for that."

It's like AN-Y-THING, AN-Y-THING! I had definitely found another official member of my Boob Dream Team!

# A Heart-to-Axilla Chat!

And then Dr. Walker, my surgeon, came in and sat for a little bit with us. You know, it's a research center. He has the time; he's not running from room to room. I mean, he's quite busy, but not in the same way. So he came in just to chat a little bit. We were chatting, then he left. And then he examined me, and he said, "You're doing fantastic."

Then I said, *[in a playful, warm tone]:* "Robert, I have spoken to my axilla!"

He said, "You have, have you?"

"Yes, I have spoken to my axilla, and she says she doesn't want to leave home."

And he smiled and said, "She does, does she?" And I said, "I have come to love you so much, and I know the scientist in you wants these nodes."

And he said, "Yes, he does, but," he says, "it's the humanist in me you're talking to, isn't it?"

I said, "Yeah."

He says, "I understand. I can't ask you to have this operation as the humanist. As the scientist, I do want those nodes."

I said, "I understand. And you know, I love you so much, I've even considered giving them to you, but I don't want to do that."

And he said, "Okay."

---

## A Heart-to-Axilla Chat!

*"Robert, I have spoken to my axilla
and she says she doesn't want to leave home.
...I know the scientist in you wants these nodes."
And he smiled and said, "Yes, he does, but it's the
humanist in me you're talking to, isn't it?"
I said, "Yeah." He said, "I understand. I can't ask
you to have this operation as the humanist."
Think about a conversation with a doctor who can put
those two things separate at the same level.*

And it was just beautiful. Think about a conversation with a doctor who can put those two things separate at the same level. Because the scientist will get a lot from those nodes for the future.

*He's an angel.*

## Sacred Hands

*Dr. Robert Walker has the healing touch*
*that you have. When he puts his hands*
*on my breast, I feel the divine.*
*I feel it. It comes through his hands.*
*The resident works on engines as a hobby, and he*
*touches my breast like he touches an engine.*
*It feels like a mechanical touch. And it's fine.*
*It's not a bad touch, but it's not a healing touch.*
*Dr. Walker has a healing touch.*
*He puts his hands on you*
*and you feel his prayer in his hands.*

He's an angel. He's a devout Mormon. I told him he's just an angel. And, you know, he has the healing touch that you have. When he puts his hands on my breast, I feel the divine. I feel it. It comes through his hands. The resident works on engines as a hobby and he touches my breast like he touches an engine. It feels like a mechanical touch. And it's fine. It's not a bad touch, but it's not a healing touch.

*It's not a nurturing touch.*

Robert Walker has a healing touch. He puts his hands on you and you feel his prayer in his hands. It is unbelievable, and I told him that. I said, "You know you are a healer and you have a healing touch." And he blushes—he blushes all the time about everything. So I am in the right place there. And, because I have such great faith in Robert, I've chosen him to put in the "port" for administering the chemotherapy. I just want Robert's hands. I want this devout man who is living with the divine.

I've been just reveling in my Boob Dream Team and the Ellis Center. That place! Those people! Because, I mean, those hands. I would have traveled the world over, to find a team like this. Where do you find a team like this? "Who" has put those people together so I would feel that it won't be chemo, it will be "therapy"? I couldn't be more grateful to have met such a powerful, wonderful doctor earlier that morning, but one from the "other world." I saw the difference between an effective medical environment, and a healing environment. It was fine, acceptable, but it wasn't a healing environment. Not a sacred environment. This is a sacred environment. They are so pleased that some-body's putting it in words and expressing it or them, because they know they have created something special.

*And you've been mirroring their excellence.*

Mirroring back to them, what they have done, and who they are. And they deserve it. "Dr. Walker," I said, "You know when you

## The Boob Dream Team

*Where do you find a team like this?*
*"Who" has put those people together so*
*I would feel that it won't be chemo,*
*it will be "therapy"?*

*...I saw the difference between an effective*
*medical environment, and a healing environment.*
*It was fine, acceptable,*
*but it wasn't a healing environment.*
*Not a sacred environment.*
*This is a sacred environment. It is just sacred.*

have your breast center, people will come from all over the world." And he said, "I hope so." And he says, "I want to franchise it. I want doctors to come and learn from us, watch us in action and then take this whole concept back home and re-create it there." I said, "Well, I'm glad they are perfecting cloning. They are going to need you there, because it's very much who you are that's creating this atmosphere."

# Cancer 101
## Enlightening...or Stifling?

So that's where I am. I've made the decision to do chemo-THERAPY in the hands of these wonderful people at Ellis. Right now I am still studying the whole thing to see which combination is the best for me. We are taking the weekend to study it thoroughly. We want to understand each drug, know what each does, know the possible side effects; not that I will need to have them, but just to know them. When I have decided which one is the one for me, I will surrender to it.

*Some people like to gather data, and feel more in control of their destiny by knowing all about what they are facing. For them it's soothing. Others like to be less focused on the specifics, and feel it helps them to maintain a positive focus. Both are open valves to well-being. Since you've made the choice to study possible side effects, it would also be a good idea to immediately begin resonating with the opposite of each symptom. If nausea is a possibility, flip to the feeling of having a very settled stomach. Just "flip it!" Resonate with that. In fact, it's a good technique for anything unpleasant that life offers. You can always find your balance by looking for the opposite, just "flip it!" Imagine what it would "feel like" to have the opposite. The wonderful thing is that you can play this mental game ahead of time, and practice several times in advance of the event. It's an energetic rehearsal. Tune-up the orchestra and let the cellular music begin!*

*[laughing]:* I can hear it now, an orchestral version of a new song called, "Just...Flip It!"

*[laughing]: There you go! Sure to quickly rise to the top of the charts. That's a good one. But back to your search for options from which to choose your "therapy." The data that you gather regarding cancer has the potential to enlighten you, but also the potential to shut you down emotionally and energetically. You may want to consider making your study as brief as possible. Study, but don't dwell on what it seems to say you are "up against." The principle still holds true that you get more of whatever it is you give your full attention to. Most people, if told that 97% will have a difficult time, identify with that, rather than the 3% that easily sail right through the process. They think they might as well face the odds. They give their power away.*

*Enlightened by*
*Studying about Cancer?*
*Or Shut Down Emotionally...*

*How does it feel?*

What I might do, is have Yumi do most of the investigating. He's excellent at doing that. I could just jump in for highlights and summaries, here and there.

*Perfect. You know how he'd love doing that for you. The scientist in him loves data.*

He'd absolutely delight in helping.

# Chapter 9

# The Alignment

## An Optional Dress Rehearsal

*Whether you are the actual chemotherapy-data-seeker or not, you can greatly benefit from using visualization techniques to enhance your experience. Well before the actual day your therapy begins, you can embellish your chemo-THERAPY experience energetically. You're such an experienced visualize-er. You might want to put your focus into a scenario like this:*

*Visualize yourself feeling beautifully nurtured by the nurses tending to you as you receive your therapy. See Yumi at your side, holding your hand and stroking your forehead. Align yourself with the "therapy in a bottle" (or bag) that you're paired with for several hours; it's your new side-kick. Acknowledge it as a healing liquid. Appreciate the wonderful "insurance" that it's providing for your body. See it as a liquid that "tidies" you up inside. Picture that drip by drip, it's delivering thousands of itty-bitty (microscopic) little maids in the cutest little outfits (maids that don't do windows, but they DO, do bodies!). See them everywhere in your body, polishing up your insides, vacuuming, fluffing, dusting, enhancing, and singing, "Happy Days Are Here Again" as they work. Yes, not only are they spiff-ing you up on the inside, but these little darlings are hosting a cellular celebration. They've brought millions of teeny-tiny balloons with them that are filled with Life Force. Looking more closely, you see that each tiny balloon has something written on it. (Grab your magnifying glass!) They say:*

"Congratulations!"                    "Happy Flying!"
        "We have Lift-Off!"    "Fueled by Joy!"
"Led by inspiration!"                    "Celestial bifocals!"
        "Angels at Work!"        "Priceless Cargo!"
"Wholeness!"                "Programmed for Self-Healing."
                "Balance."
                    ...etc.

*[laughing joyfully]:* I love the sayings!

## A Silver "Aligning"
### Visions of Good Things Dance
### in my Head during Chemotherapy

*Align yourself with the "therapy in a bottle"
that you're paired with for several hours; it's your
new side-kick. Appreciate the wonderful "insurance"
that it's providing for your body. See it as a liquid that
"tidies" you up inside. Picture that drip by drip, it's
delivering thousands of itty-bitty (microscopic)
little maids in the cutest little outfits. See them
everywhere in your body, polishing up your insides,
vacuuming, fluffing, dusting, enhancing, and singing,
"Happy Days Are Here Again" as they work.*

*I bet you'll love this, too! Each balloon is programmed to "pop" within the hour, on cue, flooding your entire body with incredible energy and well-being.*

Uhmmmm...I love that. How wonderful!

*Fast-forward to a vision of yourself having a pleasant and comfortable ride home afterwards. Enlist your invisible team (angels) to align your body, affirming that you want to feel balanced and steady—before, during and after the treatment. Continue to play it out in advance, seeing yourself comfortably going through the therapy and actually having a good time. Play it out, over and over until you can reference the therapy, and life-after-therapy, with clarity, comfort and ease. There MUST be an alignment of you—with the therapy. Oh yes, and don't forget to thank the angels and maids!*

[laughing] Absolutely! All the angels and maids. How uplifting to have all those little maids with their millions of tiny balloons! And I love the thought of balance...that's the perfect word! Balance.

*Yes. It's so thrilling to know that the human body just naturally seeks balance and is programmed for self-healing. We tend to be unconscious of all the absolute miracles that are taking place in our bodies every single minute of each day. I never tire of contemplating that piece of life. Uhmmmmm. Unseen miracles inside, even when we're having a bad day. They keep right on happening. Isn't life awesome?*

Absolutely awesome!

---

### ♥ Unceasing Cellular Miracles... Even on a Bad Day!

*It's so thrilling to know that the human body just naturally seeks balance and is programmed for self-healing. We tend to be unconscious of all the absolute miracles that are taking place in our bodies, even when we're having a bad day. They keep right on happening. Isn't life awesome?*

# *Emotional Visitors—*
# *Bearing Unexpected Gifts*

*You know, Hedy, we have these magnificent bodies, programmed for balance and self-healing. Our bodies are truly awesome! Yet, especially during life-threatening illnesses, or after a scary diagnosis, negative emotions such as worry or doubt, often cycle through our experience. They are the very things that sabotage our body's "self-balancing mechanism." Many would say, "It's only normal to worry or to be frightened. After all, we're talking about cancer here!" But the very fact that it seems only normal to have these feelings, means that they also slip quietly into our experience without triggering any warning bells—bells that would otherwise loudly ring indicating "unauthorized visitor" or "Life Force meltdown." Any negative emotions, whether stemming from a frightening diagnosis or just everyday life, still amount to disconnection from our Source Energy. Disconnection from the Kosher Choreographer! Perceived properly, these same negative emotions can be seen to bear an immediate gift; they provide a cue telling you that you've wandered off your path. The road to Health-ville and Balance-ville is straight ahead and you just temporarily veered off the road and into the bushes. There is an enormous benefit in seeing the negative emotional cues as "keys" to your well-being and good health. Become aware of how they quietly slip into your experience while disguised as "normal." Then focus on the gift they bring in the form of a "cue," rather than on trying to get rid of the negative emotions themselves.*

Yes, I love the way you describe them as "visitors coming for a little stay and bearing a house-warming gift"...and that "they weren't meant to take up residency!"

*[laughing] That's right! Accept the cue eagerly and begin to choose thoughts that feel better. Even calling any "worries"— "cues," feels better immediately. Instead of saying, "I'm worried," playfully say, "I'm cued!" The better-feeling thoughts provide an*

*immediate course correction on your journey to "where you want to be" (Balance-ville), or "whatcha-wanna-have" (fabulous health). The sooner you decide to choose better thoughts, the sooner you're accelerating your body's return to balance. You're getting out of its way.*

Yes! Yes! Gladly getting out of its way!

## "Normal" Negative Feelings?

*Many would say, "It's only normal to worry or to be frightened. After all, we're talking about cancer here!" But, the very fact that it seems only normal to have these feelings, means that they also slip quietly into our experience without triggering any warning bells— bells that would otherwise loudly ring indicating "unauthorized visitor" or "Life Force meltdown."*

*The good news is that the body is very forgiving. It's really about the RATIO of negative thoughts to positive thoughts that is most important. We're human. We're in an environment that stimulates negative thoughts in the best of us, especially when we're having a bunch of lab tests, doctor's appointments and medical procedures. Think of your momentary glitch when you received the fax containing the frightening pathology report. Talk about being wand-challenged!*

Wand-challenged for sure. We just kept making our way to the star end. We'd stay there for awhile, and then another thought would sneak in, here and there. It felt like it was something "bigger than us." What I was most thankful for, was the awareness of how much it was truly helping on all levels, when we were at the star end for even brief periods of time. We held to that simple agenda during that drive...to stay at the star end as much as we could. And so we drove, going star end—stick end—star end—stick end! Then it kind of went like, star...star...stick, star...star...star...We probably wore out several wands on that trip!

*[laughing] We'll just re-name you, "Wand-a Schleifer," sliding back-and-forth from one end of the wand to the other. You're O.K., then you're NOT O.K. You think you can do it, then you think you can't. The lab test means nothing, the lab test means this is really serious. Star end—stick end!*

*We usually have one personality inside us who is eager to keep score.*

Yes, I know that girl, the official "score-keeper."

*And we're so aware that at times like this, we "should" be more positive than ever. Our loved ones are desperately wanting us to get well. It pushes their "fear button" when they hear us becoming negative or see us wavering. Their helplessness is soothed when they hear us "talking positively." Unfortunately, situations can make us try to at least say the right words just for them. But when fear is filling our heart space, these end up being empty, disconnected words merely from our lips. **They don't count.** Your body reads your energy flow, not your lips!*

Yes, yes. We're just giving everything "lip service."

## *Positive Affirmations ... or Merely Lip Service*

*Our loved ones are desperately wanting us to get well. It pushes their "fear button" when they hear us becoming negative or see us wavering. Their helplessness is soothed when they hear us "talking positively." Your body reads your energy flow, not your lips!*

*You know, you were absolutely right when you said that the negative feelings following that scary fax report seemed so much bigger than "you." As our "perceived vulnerability" increases, **so does our resistance.** It makes us want to "push back." We try our best to shout "No" at self-defeating, scary thoughts. We engage in a game of "Push and Shout." We engage with the negativity, merely by pushing back, and the escalation begins. If we continue the game, soon we find ourselves not only engaged, but soon-to-be-married to the very partner we didn't want. We're wed to a bigger version of the initial negative emotion, the one that originally caught our eye. The sooner we remember any negativity merely as a wonderful cue (from a visitor) telling us to turn our attention towards what we really want, the sooner the negative thought will recede. By turning your attention elsewhere, you stop feeding the negative vision or issue, and it loses weight!*

Ha! You know, instead of a "support group" we could form a "Perceptual-Weight-Loss Support Group," where people come to lose weighty thoughts and lighten-up their perceptions. We could massage each other's perceptions about individual life dramas, not trying to "fix what's broken," but to help each other feel our way to a better perception. Our motto could be, "Here's another way you can look at THAT!" By the time you leave, it will look like that."

*[laughing] You're really good at this! Maybe we could give each participant a magic wand as they arrive, along with a little instruction sheet to let them know that good-feeling thoughts activate the star end. As we each took turns sharing, the rest of us could wave the stick end if they were headed in a weighty direction. (Since we're there for "perceptual weight loss!") We could have posters on the wall that say, "Well-being is Natural!" and "I am Willing to Receive!" "Joy is our Legacy!" "Lighten-up!" "I celebrate my body!" "My Spirit Soars!" I'm getting carried away here, but what a fun idea.*

It makes me want to join right now! I feel lighter just thinking about it.

*Me, too. Anyway, like I said, the good news is that it's actually the ratio of uplifting thoughts to self-defeating thoughts that's most important. The more lopsided it is, with the number of uplifting thoughts out-weighing the self-defeating thoughts, the more Life Force is freed up and the more balance is sustained.*

Uhmmm, yes. I love that. How empowering!

*So here's to the ratio that is lopsided, heavy on the happy stuff! Not just words from your lips, but words coming from your heart... a light heart that's loaded with "happy."*

Yes. Heavy on happy! I love it! We'll have to put those on the wall at the "Perceptual-Weight-Loss Support Group!"

---

### *Perceptual-Weight-Loss Support Group for Losing Heavy Thoughts!*

POSTERS FOR THE WALL:

"Well-being is natural!"     "I am willing to receive."
"Joy is Our Legacy."     "Lighten-up!"
"I celebrate my body!"     "My Spirit Soars!"
"Body fueled by uplifting visions!"
"I now reclaim my power."

# Chapter 10

# Empowerment

## Surprise! <u>YOU</u> are the Healer!

*You know, Hedy, there are so many things that are known to enhance healing: chemotherapy, radiation, medicines, prayer, herbs, acupuncture, massage, surgery, meditation, hands-on-healing, etc., to name a few. Each one has been given the credit for being the ingredient, or one in the combination of ingredients, that "totally cured cancer" in some people, some of the time; but they haven't cured all of the people, all of the time. The most important healing ingredient is actually missing from any list, unless YOU are at the very top. In other words, "YOU are the Gift!" YOU are the healer! You could say that all healing is "self-healing" because every option on that list merely supports and stimulates you to self-heal. To heal means to expand and grow into who you really are. It means opening your valve to the well-being that is natural to you. It's about embracing what is already there and has never left, even in the most awful circumstances. God never left. Your spirit never left. Linda was a prime example of one with a deteriorated body, who expanded into who she really was. Your loving touch provided a powerful touchstone for her re-alignment. Over and over you touched her with God's love.*

Absolutely! What a miracle.

*At the time of a frightening diagnosis, we want someone to "fix" us. The list of healing options acts as a soother. Healers are soothers. Whether we choose to have the cancer surgically removed, chemically eradicated, radiated, or healed energetically (prayer, laying-on-of-hands, meditation, etc.), the thought of the healing that will follow is soothing. The glitch is that we still view the healing moment as being "out there in the future" rather than in our "now." There is nothing more powerful than our "now" for really getting down to business. The soothing vision of future good health certainly opens our valve. That's admittedly a good thing. But, the part of us that keeps noticing "it isn't here yet" closes us down. Bringing the vision into our "now" is where the real power is. In other words, as I mentally embrace the vision of myself having perfect health and well-being, what choices am I making? What am I enjoying? How am I feeling? Where am I going? Going there in your mind's eye is a powerful tonic in your "now."*

You know, it makes me think of ongoing dress rehearsals before the big night. We need to find ways to "be it" in our minds, even before we have physical evidence that it has happened. Our bodies respond to the dress rehearsals right now, rather than waiting until the first curtain call on opening night.

*Exactly. No matter what we are resonating to as a healing tool, it would be more accurate to say that we are looking for something or someone to "inspire us to remember who we really are, and how magnificently we are designed." Admittedly, everything on that list has the potential to help us relax into that knowing. But, the key is to do what you've been doing on your journey. You have felt your way along as you looked for what you resonate to. You've sought the plan that you are now in alignment with. Your valve to your well-being is wide open!*

Yes. I feel such a connection with my Boob Dream Team.

*It's so common to think of ways to kill cancer, rather than to expand wellness. Killing is not our nature; even if it's cancer that's being killed. We are not natural-born killers. We are natural-born lovers. While we like knowing that cancer is gone, the perceived cellular battle in the interim is anything but a valve opener. Perceiving chemotherapy as a poison flowing through your veins is not likely to be a valve opener. It's like a lead weight around your ankles as you're attempting to fly, or that long strip of toilet paper stuck to your foot as you are making your way towards perfect health.*

*[both of us laughing]*

*[playfully]: Here, dear, let me take that off your foot!*

*[Hedy moving her head back and forth]:* Perception is everything.

*I have a dear friend who was diagnosed with cancer in her neck about 10 years ago. She had the lump removed, but decided to forego radiation and chemotherapy. Instead, she is meditating regularly and has created a very healthy style of living. Last Christmas, she wrote proudly that there was "no sign of cancer yet"! "YET!" Here we go with more toilet paper! I promptly wrote back and encouraged her to drop that "yet" right now!*

*You know, everyday, I'm more aware of the power of the spoken word. Even the word "healing" denotes something that needs to be "fixed." It actually puts your attention on "fixing," rather than on celebrating outrageously wonderful health... or celebrating the magnificence of the human body.*

I hadn't thought about that one, but you're right. It's like the stick end of the wand! Who knew? We've all used it from the beginning.

Thinking of the power of the spoken word reminds me of a phone call I received from a wonderful friend. She had just heard about my diagnosis and her voice was absolutely filled with terror. She said, in a dramatic gush, "OH, HEDY, is it true?"

And I said, "What? What?" (Truly not realizing what she could be talking about.)

She said, "Well, isn't it the Big 'C'?"

And I said, "Oh, no. It's not." "OH," she says, "Thank God. I'm so relieved. What is it?"

I said, "It's the little 'c' AND THE BIG 'ME'!"

"OH, I'M SO RELIEVED!" *[laughter]* She couldn't stop laughing after that. She just couldn't stop. You know, it just immediately diffused the power of cancer...by a mere change in the spoken word.

*How perfect!*

### It's the Big "C"!
### The power of the spoken word!

*A friend called and said dramatically, "OH, HEDY, is it true?" And I said, "What? What?" (Truly not realizing what she could be talking about.) She said, "Well, isn't it the Big 'C'?" And I said, "Oh, no. It's not." "OH," she says, "Thank God. I'm so relieved. What is it?" I said, "It's the little 'c' AND THE BIG 'ME'!"*

*She couldn't stop laughing after that. She just couldn't stop. You know, a mere change in the spoken word, and cancer was perceived as powerless.*

*You know, my friend, all along your journey, there's been a common thread in your story that has to do with your tremendous sensitivity to how you are feeling, and choosing to do what felt better. You knew not to proceed if it didn't feel right. We might want to create a new Monopoly Game that includes, "do not pass GO without feeling good, without a smile from within, without happy thoughts and a feeling of well-being."*

Exactly! A cellular board game for the perceptually-challenged!

*[laughing, hooting]: There you go! We'll take that game with us to the Perceptual-Weight-Loss Support Group!*

*If you think back about your journey, every time you found a way to think a better thought or a way to feel better, in a very real sense, it instantly welcomed the Kosher Choreographer back into your life. It opened you up for miracles and synchronicity. It was a match. It's no wonder you hooked up with this clinic, with this Boob Dream Team!*

*You know, I love comparing life to a giant Poker Game. One of the rules, naturally, is that you instantly get more of whatever you are giving your attention to. So, if you're noticing that "Life is the pits!" the Universe (or God, or Buddha, etc.) says, "I'll match that, and raise you BIG-TIME!" You win a string of things that lead you in a downward spiral in life. (And the hits just keep on coming until you change your focus.) But, when you launch into a focus on what you appreciate in life, the Universe says, "I'll match that and raise you BIG-TIME!" The better it gets, the better it gets! What most of us are after is the Royal Flush, which is living in that connected state, that Divine Flow, in every-day life.*

*When we're saying "No!" to something, we're giving that our attention and we automatically get more of that. So, it was absolutely perfect when you gave little or no attention to the doctors who "weren't what you were looking for." It was also perfect that when you resonated with Dr. Walker and others, you couldn't stop raving about the perfection. You were "Yes-ing" your way to de-light.*

*Did you get that? De-light!*

[laughing] Yes! Yes! That's great. You know, if I adored what I found, I praised it, talked about it and celebrated it. If I didn't care for what I found, I just observed, and walked on. Now, I'm off to see what combination of chemo-therapy I want to say "Yes!" to.

*The Universe is getting ready as you speak!*

## *The Letter of Empowerment*

I want to talk about the letter you sent me. I remember that day so well. I opened up the mail, and there it was. The reason this was also such a wonderful letter is that it arrived at a time when I was intuitively doing what you suggested in the letter, without naming it. Intuitively, I knew that I was going to make this a splendid adventure... and I knew that. This letter expressed what I knew to be my truth so precisely. You began:

*My Dear Magnificent Hedy,*

*This is your dear Magnificent Friend Judie, sending you a huge gift to support and cheer on the fully-empowered Hedy!* (As soon as I saw that, I thought this is just perfect and such an important point. Every once in awhile when I felt my full empowerment or happiness, I would say, "This is the weirdest thing. I just got a diagnosis of breast cancer and I feel empowered and happy." So this was wonderful to see in your letter. You continue:) *I am a self-appointed member of your support team, invisibly surrounding your heart and*

### Poker Power!

*I find life can be compared to a giant Poker Game in which you begin a new game with each new focus. The rules are that you get more of whatever you are giving your attention to. So, if you are saying that "Life is the pits!" the Universe (or God, or Buddha, etc.) says, "I'll match that and raise you BIG-TIME!" (And the hits just keep on coming until you change your focus.) But, if you say, "Life just seems to unfold for me in the most magical ways!" the Universe says, "I'll match that and raise you BIG-TIME!"*

*Yumi's* (very important) *with my heart. From miles away I am launching the energy of profound Well-being and Joy aimed straight for the two of you... don't duck!* (That was just wonderful, I could feel it whoosh right to us.)

*Here's my 'four cents' on the subject of fabulous health. In your mind's eye, picture a gorgeous, golden, magic wand... the wand of life. No assembly is required and no batteries are needed; however, it does come with a set of very clear instructions.* (I like that because you know how they say about life: It comes without a set of instructions. And the reality is it comes with a very clear set of instructions. Very simple, only three.)

1. *Use the correct end! (It's the one with the star on it.) Many people are waving the stick end in life and wondering where the magic is!*

2. *The star end is what you are wanting more of... the stick end is what you are not wanting.*

3. *You get whatever you give your full attention to... just like that!* (That is so true. You get what you give your full attention to, period. That is where all your energy is. You continue:)

*Devastating news can often make the best of us "wand-challenged" for a moment or two.* (I mean, just that expression "wand-challenged" was so marvelous.) *The trick is to limit your attention to what you are not wanting to brief periods, focusing as much attention as possible on what you DO want.* (I think that is a very important statement in the world of medicine. Doctors are vigorously searching for anything that has gone haywire in there! It's important to know what they find, but more important to know what to do with it once you've found it. It's more important to find ways to regain our emotional balance. People get "the news" about what is wrong with them and get consumed by it.)

*Absolutely.*

(You say in the letter:)
*The trick is to limit your attention to brief periods when you're focusing on what you're NOT wanting... then pour all your attention into what you DO want.* (All your attention! That is very, very important.) *The gift in a distasteful diagnosis is that it helps you quickly and clearly know what it is you are wanting...perfect health. A distasteful diagnosis provides a powerful springboard for a fabulous launch.* (Perfect imagery, perfect imagery.) *I'm aware that you are "well-launched" so-to-speak, and busy moving in the direction of a pro-active plan. All that in "wand-eze" means you are at the magical end!* (The "wand-eze" has been very funny because as soon as I read this, Yumi said, "I'll just call you Wanda-Schleifer." *[laughter]* Wanda-Schleifer. So it's been a fun thing to play with. Whenever we forget a little bit, we go, ♪♪ "Wander-Schleifer!" It's a good reminder. Your letter continues:) *However, if you bounce back and forth, engaging both ends of the wand, it neutralizes your efforts. Here are some examples of each end of the wand:*

> *"I really, really love the feeling of a healthy, vibrant body."* (star end)
>
> *"I was diagnosed with cancer."* (star end)
>
> *"I have cancer."* (stick end)
>
> *"I'm experiencing a temporary cellular challenge."* (star end)
>
> *"I love taking excellent care of my body."* (star end)
>
> *"Why me?"* (stick end)
>
> *"I'm going to beat this disease."* (stick end)

(Now, this is such an important thing because "going to beat this disease" is in our culture. It's what we think is best to do...we must fight disease big-time! We even get the feeling that it's "bigger than us" and that if we don't watch it constantly, it will over-take us when we're not looking. The truth is that there is nothing to beat. There is only to reclaim your perfect health.)

*YES! Yes, yes, yes, yes!*

(That is so important. You continue in your letter:)
*In attempting to "beat the disease," you automatically give "it" your full attention, which potentially keeps you from moving forward. Instead of trying to "beat the disease," it's more productive to celebrate life in creative new ways. For example, you exercise just because you love taking extraordinary good care of yourself and you're worth it. . . not because you have to beat a disease. There's a big difference in how your body responds between the two scenarios.*

(This next piece is brilliant.) *You come with a built-in 'wand sensor'. . . when you feel good (joyful, happy, silly, blissful, peaceful, etc.) you are at the star end. . . when you feel bad (worried, angry, frustrated, guilty, resentful, etc.) you're at the stick end. The idea is to play any game that makes you feel good, and know that on a cellular level, your cells are instantly responding with responses that lead to perfect health.*

*I love lying in bed at night and imagining that each cell in my body has a very bright light. . . I'm shimmering from head to toe. Even my eyelashes sparkle. I enjoy taking an inventory of all my internal organs and systems and seeing everything brightly lit. My heart sparkles as it beats; my blood is shimmering as it flows; my lungs sparkle as I inhale and exhale, etc. Imagine the tremendous flow of Life Force that's actually being celebrated within every cell during that vision!* (And you know, this is interesting because it's like the radioactive isotopes that they inject to outline the lesion and sentinel node. This lovely doctor, I mean this incredible presence, just injects some radioactive isotopes in the lesion. The machine has some kind of camera and there's this big picture. As you know, we saw the lesion light-up and it traveled to the sentinel node, and the sentinel node lit-up! I had tears in my eyes just to see the body the way it works like that. It works actually like that. If you put in something like Joy, the whole thing lights-up like that.)

*Absolutely. Absolutely.*

(Your letter continues:)
*I use the memory of my dog, Buttercup, to instantly reconnect me if I find myself offset by situations or events. Just having her invisibly with me... massaging the little webs between her toes (the Labrador Retriever in her), stroking the soft part of her face, etc. Bingo! I'm at the star end of the wand.* (You know, as I told you, when I was waiting for surgery, I thought, "Okay, what do I need right now that would just make me smile?" I visualized my aunt in her wig, sitting on the subway, reading the Psalms just for me. It warmed my heart and made me smile. That really came from reading your letter and that vision was just so wonderfully connecting.)

*Right, right!*

(You continue in your letter:)
*Music, art, nature, pictures I've torn from magazines, are also part of my personal "Life Force First Aid Kit." <u>Nothing</u> is ever more important than that I feel good. Only then am I allowing Life Force to enhance my body. Only then am I fully connected with my Spiritual Support Team.* (You see, this is the thing about the spiritual support team. I not only see evidence of their presence in the invisible, but actually see embodied spiritual support. I see this spiritual support coming through doctors and nurses, etc. That's who they truly are. They're Spiritual Angels in disguise!)

(Your letter continues:)

*God won't join us in blaming, worrying, fearing, etc., but waits patiently until we are willing to give our attention to loving thoughts. The only way we can truly be of any real help to others is to take care of our inner-selves first. It's like on airplanes when the emergency instructions tell us to put on our own oxygen mask before assisting those around us.*

*I send you and Yumi fabulous insight, strength and the knowledge that this whole scenario contains a huge gift...wrapped in the package of breast tissue.* (That's just unbelievable. I've begun to use that expression, "wrapped in a package of breast tissue.") *Along with whatever medical or surgical intervention you are "inspired" to choose...* ("Inspired" is the key word. "Inspiration" is so important. Yes, I'm inspired to do this; no, I'm not inspired to do that...Ohh, there's one that's just right for me. You know, one of the things I was inspired to do was to stop listening to my phone messages. I haven't responded. I have felt inspired to maintain my positive focus above all else. I had quickly found that many of the well-meaning messages were only disconnecting me. They were messages coming from the stick end of the wand. Louise has just taken over that whole task for me. STAYing focused is the key.)

## A Gift

*...This whole scenario contains a huge gift, wrapped in breast tissue. ...Along with any medical or surgical intervention you are inspired to choose, find every creative way to choose and celebrate wellness and wholeness.*

(Your letter continues:)
*...find every creative way to choose and celebrate wellness and wholeness. Dance the medical dance only*

*long enough to gather beneficial data and then twirl off into what you are wanting.* (Yes, I even danced the Lumpectomy Dance! And you know, in dancing that dance I really welcomed the event and created a smoooooth experience.)

•

(Your letter continues:)

*You never benefit by being at war or fighting against what you are not wanting. This is the dance of remembrance...the dance that awakens you more fully to the truth of your being. It has a profound rhythm to it. Listen for the beat of life. Watch for every possible creative way to put your attention fully on joy, health and life.* (That is beautiful. Oh, Judie! It's such an inspiring statement. Do you hear me? I'm just going to read this again. That sentence really jumped out of the page.) *This is the dance of remembrance...the dance that awakens you more fully to the truth of your being. It has a profound rhythm to it...listen for the beat of life...watch for every possible creative way to put your attention fully on health and life.* (Profound. Absolutely inspired!)

*And...when friends are anxious to help and ask if there's just anything they can do? say, "Yes! Please take one or two minutes here and there each day to imagine me enjoying my perfect health and well-being. Associate the mere mention of my name with words like 'healthy, vibrant, amazing, steady, fabulously-alive, strong, and sparkling.' And hold thoughts of me paired with tremendous cellular harmony, cellular giggles, sparkling light in every cell, and Life Force flowing abundantly throughout my body...big-time! That is the greatest gift you could give me!" (Unless they also do windows!) Count on me for doing exactly that (but not the windows).*

*There is enormous love here for you! Call me anytime you want me to rattle off more of the same to you. I love you!*

*In Joy, Judie*

## Is There Just Anything I Can Do?
### (Giving the Greatest Gift!)

*When friends are anxious to help and*
*ask if there's just anything they can do? say,*
*"Yes! Please take one or two minutes here and*
*there each day to imagine me enjoying*
*my perfect health and well-being. Associate the*
*mere mention of my name with words like*
*'healthy, vibrant, amazing, steady, fabulously-alive,*
*strong, and sparkling.' Hold thoughts of me paired with*
*tremendous cellular harmony, cellular giggles, sparkling*
*light in every cell, and Life Force flowing abundantly*
*throughout my body...big-time!*
*That is the greatest gift you could give me!"*
*(Unless they also do windows!)*

I have truly carried your letter everywhere with me and read it over and over. When I was wand-challenged Thursday, I read it again. I also made myself a little file that says "inspiration," and I not only put a copy of your letter in it but also the other thing you sent me with thoughts on how to go to a doctor's appointment and still maintain my connection. I just read it all again. Reading these things instantly help me to remember where it's really at. I mean, sometimes I just get knocked off my center for a little while.

*Sure. It can even come from sources like the evening news or a magazine. It can really sneak up on you!*

I ran into this woman the other day (whom I know very well). She said, "What are you doing here at the hospital?"

I said, "I have a diagnosis blah-bedy blah..." and I told her my story. She said, "And are you going to do chemo?"

And I said, "I don't know." I had just come out of that doctor's office and I just said, "I don't know yet. I'm just waiting for inspiration about it."

She said, "Oh, yes. Chemo's a baaad thing, you know. It can leave you with side effects for the rest—of—your—life." And she began to talk, and I could just feeeel the energy draining from me. She frightened me.

Later, in the car, I said to Yumi, "Oh, gosh, maybe I'd better call this woman about the side effects for the rest of your life." And Yumi says, "<u>No way</u> are you calling this woman about the side effects for the rest of your life."

He says, "She's not talking about **you!**" "Oh," I said, "Right... I remember...I am the Magnificent Wanda-Schleifer." *[laughing]*

*Invisible Drain-o...followed by "Wanda Schleifer." And we have re-connection!*

*That's fabulous. What perfect timing. Yumi tossed you the star end of the wand! Imagine fast forwarding to a time when you are looking back at this journey, and <u>you</u> come across someone who is reeling over a frightening diagnosis. Perhaps they've recently been diagnosed, just like you were in that story. But instead of joining the fear, you give them a touchstone through your vision of well-being that helps them feel their way to higher ground... higher ground where they can breathe easier and steady them-selves. You tell them about the magic wand and your real name of Wanda Schleifer! The two of you laugh together at it all. What a difference. Instead of sucking them dry, you've soothed them into their spiritual connection.*

Absolutely. There's such a difference.

*It's so common for people to want to share what they think they really know a lot about. After they've survived months of fright-ening drama and perceived vulnerability, they've amassed a lot of data regarding it all. They think it's helpful to pass it on. Unfortunately, what they've become experts about is "fear" and all the ins-and-outs of fighting disease...instead of knowing about the celebration of the body, and health and life.*

*Consequently, they unwittingly hand the stick end of the wand to others. They attempt to use fear as a common denominator in order to bond with someone who has a similar diagnosis. But, if they're lucky, along comes "Wanda Schleifer" marching to a refreshingly new beat! She tucks an enormous gift into even the briefest encounter and massages their feelings of empowerment and their ability to focus on well-being.*

## Invisible Draino!

Well, I ran into this woman the other day
(whom I know very well). She said,
"What are you doing here at the hospital?"
"I have a diagnosis blah-bedy blah..."
And I told her my story. She said, "And are you
going to do chemo?" And I said, "I don't know."
I had just come out of that doctor's office and
I just said, "I don't know yet. I'm just waiting
for inspiration about it." She said, "Oh, yes.
It's a baaad thing. It can leave you with side effects for
the rest—of—your—life." And she began to talk, and I
could just feeeel the energy draining from me.

Yes! Pass the star end of the wand please. *[laughing]* I must, however, confess to you something that is very interesting. Some of the time I have responded in a way that I have found a little embarrassing. I call this version of me "the brazen hussy."

Sometimes, when I acutely felt people's fear as they greeted me...like, *[in a cascading tone]*:
"Oh Hedy,

    **How**

        **are**

            **yooooou?"**

(Said in such a sad tone, reflecting, "Oh you poor, poor thing...tell me all the bad that has happened to you.")

Well, in being determined not to pair up with that even for a minute, I found myself going overboard with positive-ness. You and I both know, that's not really being at the star end of the wand. To be honest, I was really being a little bit cocky about it.

*Well, admittedly there's a bit of a "push" against their sadness in your response, but it's a good beginning.*

Yes, it's a good beginning.

*And, you know how to access better-feeling thoughts from that beginning. The first step is always in being sensitive to how you feel. The "cockiness" didn't feel like authentic up-liftment; it smacked of a partially counterfeit moment.*

Yes, I felt a little embarrassed about my cockiness. But you know what? I look at it today and say, "It's better to have been cocky, than to join their fear and gloom-and-doom—and then have to rise up out of all <u>that</u>." The second version would have been a deeper fall into the "hole of where I don't want to be."

*And, you've just made a perfect beginning statement for "feeling your way back" to your center. That's precisely how it's done. You notice you feel uncomfortable, reach for a thought that feels better, and it attracts yet another thought that feels even better. In moments, we have a "re-centered Hedy."*

Yes! So I'm just going to be very forgiving for my brazenness and cockiness.

*Absolutely. It's early training in a new arena.*

—My early training.

*Cockiness can temporarily serve as your training wheels. It's a way of steadying yourself as you run smack into the fear-based realities of how others view cancer, until you can find a more authentic response. Once you've truly regained your balance about this issue, similar comments will sail right on by. That was how you handled these encounters in the beginning. More and more you'll become so steady that you will respond to anything similar with a genuine sense of allowing. You can even rehearse for that moment in advance. For instance, imagine speaking in a soft and even manner that reflects your empowerment, your centered-ness. You speak in a manner that's so centered that they are swept up in it. Upon hearing their fear, perhaps you say something like, "Oh, I understand what you're feeling, but I have to tell you that, in terms of being healthy, I am in a better spot regarding my body than ever before. I'm actually healthier than I've ever been." It won't be your words that touch them as much as the music in your heart, as you speak your truth. You'll have set your own tone that resonates from your Core, and they'll feel it. "Oh, my," they'll say, "Oh, I see. I really see." In fact, their fear won't even qualify as a button on your dashboard in life. It won't be an option on this latest model of YOU!*

Uhmmm, you're absolutely right. It will pass right through.

*I'm curious. You are so familiar with the unhealthy-ness of carrying old hurts, regrets, judgements, unresolved painful moments, etc. How do you personally process things like that?*

Where do I put that to let it drain?

*Yeah.*

You know, I am so fluid in my life now. If I need to cry, I cry. If I need to laugh, I laugh. If I need to be scared, I'm scared. It's not the joining of the fear, it's more just a feeling it and letting it move on through.

*That's what I'm talking about. It doesn't stay.*

It doesn't stay. It just flows. Like when I shook following the surgery, I just allow it to flow right on through, without resisting it, until it disappears.

*Fabulous! What a great approach. Because, you know, whether we're feeling old pain, new pain, terrible situations on the evening news, or reeling from a frightening diagnosis, it all amounts to stifled Life Force. It's a cellular challenge for the entire time you hold that perspective. Your willingness to let it flow right on through is fabulous.*

Absolutely.

*I personally think that the reason this works so well for you is that your focus during the process is on the release, allowing whatever-it-is to surface and leave. Focusing on the pain itself would make it an unending cycle.*

Yes, the focus is on allowing it to pass. I surrender to it and let it go right on through without resisting.

*You know that old saying, "What you resist, persists!" It pays to find any method that lets it go. Take death, for instance. It seems like a cruel set-up to realize that, when we're grieving over the loss of someone dear, we're also blocking all spiritual support at the same time. We're at the stick end of the wand in our grief; all, while begging for peacefulness and for the pain to cease. Peacefulness can't come to us until we're willing to shift our focus.*

*When my dog Buttercup died, I would have paid you $5000 to have her back for even an hour. And then I would have paid you again for just one more hour. I knew deep inside, that she was actually alive-and-well "on the other side," and had merely changed form. Somehow, that just didn't help. I just wanted her back. I was in tremendous pain. And to make matters worse,* *being "stuck in grief" had me feeling like I was also flunking "Spirituality 101" and failing to "Walk my Talk." I was judging myself, big-time. (There was my cue!) Gradually though, my focus shifted from "wanting her back," to "wanting to feel better." I remembered to ask my favorite "What's another way I can look at this?" question. Well, the good news is that I got my Buttercup back! My new vision led me to see clearly that I could mentally choose to be "with her" instead of "without her." I spent time mentally stroking her cheek and rubbing the web between her toes, as I had done a million times before. The pain stopped instantly. I was at the star end of the wand once again. (A thrilling slide!) You can't be at both ends of the wand simultaneously. It's one or the other. Now Buttercup goes everywhere with me. Every time I throw her a stick (end of the wand), she brings me back the star end. She has given new meaning to the term "retriever." She retrieves my center any time I lose it for even brief periods.*

Uhmmm. That's a fabulous story. What a gift she gave you!

*And continues to give me! It meant that a year later when my Mom died, I was able to skip the grief process entirely, and instantly "be with her" instead of "without her." I was extremely close to my mother and adored her. Just when she passed, I immediately felt my heart expand. It was what my friend Esther Hicks calls being "hugged from the inside out!" My mother was hugging me big-time. If I had been closed down in grief I would not have been able to feel this inner hug. I've continued right-on enjoying her presence in my life every single day. She's merely changed form. It's a rich experience and a powerful perspective.*

Absolutely. You're "with her" instead of "without her." How powerful.

*It's like a soothing salve for the soul! It's a choice we can make. Even though we're more familiar with grieving, I feel that this is the version that's natural for us. This is how we were meant to process life transitions. Until we move through the grief, we lose on several levels. We can't hear guidance, our Life Force is stifled, and it's impossible for us to connect with any loved one who made his or her transition—because they are vibrating in pure joy. We're not a match! We can't hear them or connect with them. Connection is a sacred choice. Each time I find a creative way to feel my way to a better spot, it seems to expand that ability for the next occasion. It's like exercising a muscle...it gets easier and easier to think a better thought about life scenarios. You might call it "Creative Perceptual Aerobics." It frees the cement from my wings. Simultaneously my cells are "humming" with newly freed Life Force.*

I love that..."Creative Perceptual Aerobics"...do you need a cute little leotard for that?

*[laughing] That's the good part. You can even do this aerobics class—naked!*

*You know, my friend, I have watched you, and listened to you carefully ever since you were first diagnosed. Not once have I felt that you were just trying to be a Pollyanna about receiving an official notice of a "cellular challenge." Not once did I feel that you were in denial. You just didn't spend time dwelling on the possibilities that didn't serve you well. You focused upon the solution and not the problem. That's how we are meant to operate. We are meant to see what it is we are not wanting, and then let heaven pour through us as we focus on what we are wanting. You found things to appreciate (pieces of heaven) while collecting all the things that could be beneficial to your experience.*

*At times when you were "wand-challenged," you noticed it, and promptly began feeling your way back to the star end. I guess I just want to end today's session by saying that God is very, very proud. She salutes you.*

She salutes us. She salutes us. *[giggles]*

# My Invisible Buttercup, "Retriever Extraordinaire"

When my dog Buttercup died, I would have
paid you $5000 to have her back for even an hour.
And then I would have paid you again for just
one more hour. I knew deep inside, that she was
actually alive-and-well, and had merely changed form.
Somehow, that just didn't help. I wanted her back.
I was in tremendous pain. And to make matters worse,
being "stuck in grief" had me feeling like I was also
flunking "Spirituality 101" and failing to "Walk my Talk."
I was judging myself, big-time. (There was my cue!)
Gradually, my focus shifted from "wanting her back,"
to "wanting to feel better." I remembered to ask
my favorite "What's another way I can look at this?"
question. Well, the good news is that I got
my Buttercup back! My new vision led me to see clearly,
that I could mentally choose to be "with her" instead of
"without her." I spent time in my mind, stroking her
cheek, and rubbing the webs between
her toes as I had done a million times before.
The pain stopped instantly. I was at the star end
of the wand once again. (A thrilling slide!)
Now Buttercup goes everywhere with me.
Every time I throw her a stick (end of the wand),
she brings me back the star end. She has given new
meaning to the term "retriever." She retrieves
my center any time I lose it for even brief periods.

# Chapter 11

# Rituals and Readiness

## *The Circle of Fear*

You know, Yumi did an amazing job of studying tons of information about chemotherapy, and we reviewed it together. Then one morning I awoke absolutely inspired as to which chemotherapy "cocktail" I wanted, and the precise number of doses that was right for me. It just came to me like a gift. It was so wonderfully liberating. I felt absolutely empowered. I also felt moved to plan a ritual ceremony that would totally welcome this "therapy," and set the stage. My inspiration to do a ritual actually came from reading Jean Shinoda Bolen's book, *Close to the Bone*. In it, she mentions a ritual for chemotherapy. And I thought, "Wow, I really would like to do that." I'd like to do a ritual for welcoming chemotherapy.

A dear friend had come to visit that same morning, and I was crying tears of joy and saying, "I have just gotten my answer. I'm going to do chemotherapy, and I'm going to do it four times with these two drugs, <u>and</u>... I'm going to do a little ritual to usher me into this new journey." "Oh," she said, "That is wonderful, and we need to be part of it."

*There's such a surge in Life Force when you come to an inspired decision. You, the fully-connected "You," had made Your choice.*

**My** choice. And, later when I told the radiation oncologist, he said, "Oh, four times C-A, that's exactly the best treatment for this situation."

*Yes, yes.*

And then, as you know, I didn't have to do a thing for the ceremony; friends saw to all the details. Such incredible women showed up, beautiful women I've known for years, including you! I adore these women. In many cases, we've been together through various crises, through thick-and-thin, Batmitzvah's and Barmitzvah's, births and deaths, health and disease, marriage and divorce, graduations, etc. Several had been clients of mine over the years.

*It was so clear that they were eager to return some of the loving support you had so generously given to them, for such a long time. They were really "there" for you. It was very touching. It was now your turn to receive, and they were eager to play their important supporting roles. It feels so good to have "something" to do to be truly helpful at a time when such a feeling of helplessness prevails.*

Yes, it was very touching. The surprise was that this turned out to be a group of women filled with fear about my impending journey. It was a circle of fear. I was so thankful that YOU were there!

*Many just weren't skilled yet in sending invisible, positive, energetic gifts without the fear. They did what they knew best. In several cases, it seemed that your journey suddenly provided an incredible mirror, reflecting their own pain from the past, back to them.*

Yes! Yes.

*I think this just hit too close to home. Just the word "cancer" quickly fired up their perceived vulnerability, and sent up emotional flares illuminating their own "stuff." They had accidentally slid to the stick end of the wand while trying to be of enormous help.*

That's it. Perceived vulnerability.

*You know, many of those women have known each other for years. While I knew some of them, I was essentially a newcomer to the core group. I was also, as you know, totally unfamiliar with Jewish tradition, and really looking forward to what I was sure would be a beautiful Jewish-flavored ceremony. I was eager to play a quietly supportive role, invisibly adding my joy to the day and allowing others there to lead the way. I thought, I'll just quietly bless, blend, and enjoy the ceremony. Yes, I'll quietly blend. Right! Little did I know, how impossible it would be for me to cooperate with my own agenda! Me...quiet? What a laugh. The minute I arrived, I could feel the heaviness of the energy in the room. Conversations seemed so—"tastefully solemn"...I don't do "solemn." This was such a shift from the hours and hours I had spent with you laughing about "life after diagnosis!" and hearing story after story about your tenaciousness for joy in your journey. This just didn't seem to fit. Soon, I also felt as if I didn't fit either. (That was my cue!) "Just blend," I thought... "Find things to appreciate and just blend." I knew that I had to get my "oxygen mask in place" first, if I was to stand any chance of lifting the energy in the room. I began appreciating the sincere desire each of these women had to help you.*

Yes...appreciation is such a powerful valve-opener.

*Before you came down to join us, we had formed a circle, and were feeling our way along with introductions and greetings. I was still telling myself to "be quietly supportive and blend." I continued to find things to appreciate. But, the minute Louise began speaking to the group, I soon found that I couldn't keep still. She*

*announced that, "Tomorrow Hedy is going for her chemotherapy."
I interjected softly, "She wants to refer to it as 'therapy.'" She
continued on, quite willing to call it "therapy," and talking about
your upcoming journey. Then she asked us to think of our most
challenging, darkest moments, and come up with a word or
words that would be the strength or inspiration we derived from
that experience. We were each to write the words on a tiny little
square of colored paper that would be given to you for your
journey. You would then have them to help you, during challenging times ahead. Well, I instantly felt resistance inside. I mean,
I could feel the energy drop further as this group of women simultaneously referenced painful, dark moments from the past.
I thought, "I can't do this. I don't want to play this game!"
I focused instead on the fact that it was a very sweet idea, and
full of well-meaning intentions. I jotted down an inspiring word
on my piece of colored paper, without taking a mental trip to the
"Land of Challenge." I went straight to the nearby "Land of Joy
and Uplift-ment." It's just a personal preference. Once again I
thought, "Blend, just blend!" I noted that this was just a different style of helpfulness.*

That's amazing. *[laughing]* It's a different style, and it's also
taking the long route!

*Absolutely. We joined hands in the circle and Louise proceeded to
have us reflect on ways in which we were going to help "heal our
Hedy." Suddenly, a voice rose up in me that I just could not
squelch. Still holding hands in the circle, I said, "I'd like to add
something here, if I may." (I had this wild dialogue going on
inside me...the 'other voice' still saying 'just blend!' and this new
one saying, 'I must speak up...I must speak up!' These conflict-
ing inner agendas prompted a simultaneous vise-like grip of the
poor women's hands I was holding on each side of me.) I continued,
"When we think of healing, we often think of it, not from the point
of embracing health, but in terms of needing to 'fix' something.
From that standpoint, the word doesn't serve us well. It basically*

*means that we are joining the problem with our focus and our energy. Rather than 'fixing what we think is broken,' healing is about embracing what is natural to us all along. It's about reclaiming the truth about ourselves and reclaiming our power. The greatest thing we can do for Hedy is not to try to fix or heal her, but to raise our eyes to see her in perfection. See her radiance. See her totally whole and filled with aliveness. Celebrate life with her and speak about joy, strength, and well-being." Everyone listened thoughtfully and seemed to truly care about what I had proposed.*

*While still reeling from the bold and outspoken girl inside me who had insisted on being heard (part of me wished I had left her home!), the group moved on to join in singing a Hebrew song. Over and over we sang the lyrics in Hebrew. The English translation was, "Please, God, please, heal her, please." Again, it was a beautiful gesture, but I still couldn't get comfortable cycling a repeated plea for healing...I would have preferred to sing a song that celebrated all that we are and our strength! One that celebrated the divine in each of us. A song perhaps pairing all of us with strength, "cellular confidence," balance, wholeness and Joy, etc.*

You know, we'll have to look for a song that does just that! Or...maybe even compose one ourselves and teach it to everyone. I've already made one up to go with my "lumpectomy dance." *[laughter]*

*Now you're talkin'! Well, by the time I had discouraged the use of their favorite "h" word (healing), everyone became over-sensitized to the word "healing" for the rest of the ceremony. By the time you joined the group, they were stumbling every time they tried to express themselves without using the word "healing,"...or they used it, apologetically. Part of me felt as if I had ruined the whole ceremony. (Oops! Slam. Valve closed!)*

The amazing thing was that while you were feeling uncomfortable about expressing our shared viewpoints to this group, at that same moment I was upstairs asking for an angel to focus this ceremony on Joy, empowerment, and ease, etc. You turned out to be my angel! For awhile, I had been rehearsing what I could say to let them know how I was embracing this event; that it's an adventure for me, and how the choice for (chemo) "therapy" had been divinely guided, and that I am so fully alive with this journey, and that I'm in awe with how it's unfolded. But then I thought, with you there, it's going to be handled. I mean you were my angel once again on that day. If you hadn't been there, I'm sure I would have slid back to being nine years old, and would have been enveloped by this enormous room of fear. For just brief moments I slipped into feeling like a little child, feeling BIG FEAR around "little me." The majority of the time I relaxed because you were there, and ultimately I left very happy. I was translating and translating as people in the circle expressed from their hearts. They'd say what they felt and I'd silently say, "What they really mean is...blah, blah, blah." You really did as much as you could to give most of them their first lesson in the "language of well-being."

At any rate, at some point I was told that they were ready for me to come downstairs. I started going down those steps and, Judie, the energy in that room was so, uhm, **heavy**...I didn't want to go into that circle!

*I'll say it was heavy.*

Heavy. It was so heavy. It didn't feel like it was a circle for me. It felt like it was a circle to hold their fear, but it wasn't a circle for me. *[in a "Groucho Marx" style]:* The last thing I wanted to do was to step into it! *[laughing]*

As I went a little further down and I saw everyone standing in a circle, solemnly singing in Hebrew, I couldn't hold back... that's when I just got the giggles! It was a combination of embarrassment and just the only way I knew to break the heaviness. And so, when I came inside of the circle, I just laughed and laughed and laughed, and it broke up the song and changed the atmosphere. That's when I teased, *[again in "Groucho Marx" style]:* "All this ceremony! I'm only going to Sara—sota!"

*That really was effective. Your giggles were the perfect antidote.*

*I'll never forget how quickly you realized that I had been offering a "perceptual massage" to the group, prior to your entrance. And the way you leaned forward in the circle so that you could see me (grinning from ear to ear), and said in that appreciative and playful tone, [sing-song]: ♪♪ "Ohhhhhh, you've—been—talking—to—them!" ♪♪ That was great. However, I was still admittedly uncomfortable, and felt as if I had put a damper on the ceremony. (Valve closed!) I continued to participate in the best way I could and secretly planned a personal exit at the earliest opportunity. I also thought I'd stop for a big fat hamburger on the way home—comfort food! (And a valve opener! Fast-food can be soul-food, in some instances!) It would be days later before I would hear your personal version of the event and know the perfection in my participation.*

Isn't that just amazing? And here I was, so grateful that you helped smooth the way and guide it towards what I was wanting and needing.

*Just the anticipation of comfort food, put me in a slightly better spot. I was able to get on with enjoying the rest of the ceremony. I loved the part where you were lying on the floor in the middle of our circle, proudly showing off your new black "sports bra!" You looked so radiant, holding that long-stemmed red rose, your head cradled in the lap of your dear friend Elizabeth, surrounded by women who adore you. I loved watching, as we each took turns anointing you with oil. I deliberately looked for other things to appreciate about the Hebrew song we were once again singing for that portion. Over and over we sang softly, "Please, God, please, heal her please." "Ana El na, refah na lah..." (the lines Moses cried to God when Miriam was stricken with leprosy). This time, my attention was drawn to the beautiful way each woman anointed you with oil, and how sweetly everyone was singing the song. I just translated it to mean they truly were celebrating your radiant health. I was admittedly feeling better.*

[laughing] Yes. Thank goodness. You could tell that some of the energy had shifted a bit by then.

*Yes. And I also thought that they seemed to be singing from a little different "spot" inside them. I loved the part where we each blessed bottled water that you would take with you to drink, and intentionally energized stones for you to keep with you. (I filled the stones with Joy, balance and wholeness.) Others had brought tapes of guided meditations for your "healing ☺ journey."*

Yes, and you know, I found later that so many of the guided visualizations were still designed to lead you down a visual path of "pushing against" or fighting cancer. Tapes that were created by some of the best known professionals in the field! The gesture of the gift was wonderful, but the actual tapes were not what I resonated to. That's why, later, I asked you to create tapes just for me, that would say it in the way that kept me at the star end of the wand.

*I agree. Guided visualizations that are designed to empower us are priceless. You just have to be aware that there are many differ-ent styles on the market. I had such fun personalizing the ones I made for you.*

*Along with the tapes people gave you, you received so many wonderful gifts as tokens of their love and support for you.*

Yes, such wonderful gifts!

*The rest of the event seemed to grow increasingly lighter. Your sense of humor and playfulness throughout it all really helped.*

Yes. I sort of picked through the mix, and accepted the parts I resonated to.

*You know, I loved the way Louise was unceasing in finding every possible way to help smooth your journey. She had each of us bring food dishes we had prepared for you so that none of you would have to cook, and you could just focus on feeling good. Later she delivered the food to your condo where it would be waiting when you arrived. What a friend!*

Yes, you know she even handled all my telephone messages so that I wouldn't be overwhelmed. She gave me a few that she knew I'd want to handle personally and handled the rest herself. I could put all my energy into focusing on health. She's the one who thought of doing that for me. We've known each other so long, and have been so close; she was perfect for fielding everything. She kept messages going over e-mail, to keep everyone up to date on my journey, and asking for their good thoughts and prayers. It was just incredible support from her... and also from these women, on this day.

*You know, now I see even more perfection to the event, as we're looking back weeks later. The bottom line is that many, in this group of women whom you absolutely treasure, didn't have a clue as to how to speak to you so that you could more easily move forward, so that they wouldn't pull you down. It turned out to be one of those times where you think you're showing up for one thing, and the gift ends up being a totally different thing. You perceived it as a ritual to welcome this next part of your journey. It wasn't in the form you had pictured. But it absolutely "set the tone" for the kind of support you would appreciate and resonate to during the months to come. We just had to get their valves open and their "Authentic Selves" front and center. It seemed that "solemn-ness" and "fear" was initially their way of being authentic during the event. After all, their dear friend had been diagnosed with CANCER! This ritual was about getting them familiar with the note you were singing, so they could sing that note with you during your journey. The ritual was about you saying, "Hmmmm...here's my note! All together now, Hmmmm!"*

Yes! Yes!

*Thank heaven you giggled and laughed! The good news was, (as you and I would find out in the weeks to follow) that this very same group loved you so much that they would gradually be willing to re-invent themselves, as the true empower-ers and uplift-ers that you wanted all along. One by one they would eagerly show up sporting a new language of well-being. They would write different words, speak different words and refer to your entire experience in a whole new way. Gradually, they could think of you, and your diagnosis of cancer, and keep their valves open at the same time. Joy? Peace? Spiritual Confidence? Cellular confidence? Eagerness for this journey? All of that paired with a diagnosis of cancer? Who'd have thought it! And that all began at this ceremony. Now THAT was quite a ritual!*

Yes! Yes!

*All we were asking on the day of the ceremony was that each one change their entire orientation to life and speak a new language. That's all!! [laughing] They rose to the challenge. The pay-off in every direction was much greater than if we had just kept quiet and had not massaged their original version of the ceremony. Yes, thank goodness you dared to laugh! Giggle power!*

I love that, "giggle power!" You're absolutely right. It was a powerful beginning. We just had to go back to basics and then begin again. It was a refresher course in "Spiritual Alignment 101"!

## A Detour to Lake Barf
### (After the first "therapy")

I will never forget my first evening after having the very first dose of (chemo) therapy. You know, I also had the minor surgery to insert what they call a "port" that would be used to administer each treatment. So I had general anesthesia, and then the "therapy." It all seemed to go smoothly. Nobody mentioned that I should rest, so we just did our thing. You know, I ate, we hung around and visited with the staff, and two or three hours later we left for the condo which friends had prepared for us at Cocoa Beach.

Yumi was driving the Lexus, Yigal was in the back seat and I was in the front. At some point—it seemed like out of nowhere, I began vomiting. It was a kind of sensation that I had never experienced before. Not just vomiting...my whole body was in a revolution, and there was just no stopping it when it decided to come up!

*I'll say. It sounded very impressive from this end, when you called me on your car phone! You'd be talkin' one minute, and vomiting the next! [sympathetic laughter]*

Ahh. I mean, every part of my body was in revolt. It was my stomach, it was my cells, and it was the treatment. It was a major revolt.

*Major objection.*

MAJOR objection! Aah! And I was just vomiting and vomiting and vomiting. You know, and we had those suppositories, but we didn't know if we should put them in because I'd already taken this pill and that pill—anyway, we were just really helpless. I felt powerless. I felt overpowered. And the Lexus was filled with vomit. I mean it was just everywhere. *[laughter]* It was on my pants. It was on the floor. It was on the doors. It was on the dash. It was on Yumi's clothes. Because, you know, it wasn't the kind of vomit where you politely open the window or door. I was like Mt. Vesuvius! It was just all over.

*A sneak attack!*

Yes! And the interesting thing was, after each episode, I knew I wasn't done! I mean, we were already sitting in this pool of vomit, and I wasn't done yet! *[laughing]* We had pulled over to this lake, which we later named "Lake Barf." Days after all this, Yumi confessed that he was certain that the Lexus had literally been "totaled," and we'd never be able to return it to normal. But at this point, his only concern was finding relief for me.

We had tried to call the hospital on the car phone, tried the doctor, you know, couldn't reach anybody we knew at that hour. We got some other doctor who was sort of impatient with our nervousness and helplessness. And, finally we thought to call you. I mean, it was like we really needed somebody in the picture and you were the angel that answered our call. You literally "talked me through to the comfort of my bed," over an hour later.

*The interesting thing was that normally, I wouldn't have even been available at that time. As it happened, I was sitting right next to the telephone, reading something. It was perfect timing.*

Absolutely orchestrated! We asked the nurse in you, "Should we put in the suppository for vomiting?" and you said, "Yes." So we stopped at a 7-11, did that, and we came back. And the fact that I knew you'd be there...that your voice was going to be in the car when we returned was very important. It filled the car with that atmosphere of calm, delight, hope, and the knowing that there is a wonderful light at the other end of the tunnel. Since we had you on the speaker phone, all three of us were soothed with your wonderful voice. You provided a steady stream of guided imagery...enjoying all the good things in advance. It was like a friend of mine once said, you helped me to "borrow a dance from the future, when there wasn't anything here now to dance about!" I said, "I just want to be in my bed at the condo now." And you quickly said, "Well, let's go there right now! Lean back, and in your mind's eye, see the three of you pulling into the parking place at your condo...opening the door and ascending the stairway to the master bedroom." In your soft meditative voice, telling me (while talking over static at your end), "You're now slipping into the silky percale sheets and relaxing into the support of the mattress beneath you. You take a nice long, deep breath. As you settle down, you can hear the sound of the waves on the shore…you can feel the coolness of the sheets on your body…you can see right through the ceiling to the stars above, and easily breathe the cool night air."

And, I was visually, right with you! Yes! I thought—"I can see right through the ceiling!" I was attempting to really allow myself to step into that fully. It sustained me for long periods of time… And then the next thing you knew, I'm motioning for Yumi to pull over, while I vomit again! Then we would begin our journey once again with your "visions of well-being" serenading, calming and soothing the three of us. Yigal, who has never met you, said, "Mom, I'm in love with this woman! I'm in love with this woman." *[laughing]* The whole time…every time we'd hear your voice, "I'm in love with this woman."

To have your voice for over an hour, filling our car, steadying all three of us. You never wavered. It was soft, it was loving, it was supportive, it was angelic. I mean, it was just holding me through that experience. It was my salvation. That's what carried me. You know, Yumi was there, Yigal was there, but that voice, your voice. And your energy, as you were sending these visions. You were sending healing energy right over the telephone!

*Oh…you caught me!*

We finally arrived at the condo and immediately called you back so you could continue this wonderful imagery another 30 minutes, the time when I could take the next dose of medication. Thank goodness that as the night progressed, I steadily became more settled.

You know, I learned an important lesson here. I had found the perfect cocktail for me, and the perfect place to have it administered, and the perfect staff to be at my side, BUT…I truly think that I still perceived this "therapy" as somewhat of a "poison" being put into my sacred body. I really didn't welcome it. I tolerated it. And, I underestimated the collective energy that is paired with even the subject of "chemotherapy," as the result of millions of people fearing it and hating to have it. There's a huge emotional package invisibly attached to the treatment. I unwittingly lined up with the fear instead of the blessing it was providing. My body is so sensitive...and I am so sensitive. No wonder there was a major revolt!

*As you put it, your body is so "conscious!"*

Absolutely. The good news is that this was the first and last time I would have this problem following my therapy. Even though each dose that followed was stronger than the previous one, I did better and better each time. I learned to align my thoughts and align my body, in a way that I would actually welcome each treatment. An important part of that alignment was listening to the guided meditations you recorded for me as I was receiving each dose. It just helped me to continue to align...continue to align... and continue to welcome this therapy. With each of the following doses, I was stronger, and had an increasingly better appetite. The power of the mind is absolutely awesome!

*The power of alignment!*

## The Right of Passage

This was also a very important time for our son Yigal...it was the right of passage for him. There were two things he did. One was that he knew "all is well," and he kept knowing that at the deepest level of his being. He sees his mother vomiting all over the place after (chemo) therapy, and his father (who is always on top of everything) is absolutely LOST about what to do for her. And throughout it all, this 28-year-old young man was just totally connected to Source. "All is well." He knew it. He kept holding steadily to that.

The other thing he did was that he cleaned the car in the middle of the night, so that his dad would wake up and find a clean Lexus. Well, Judie, what that young man had to clean! I mean, a toilet is nothing compared to what he had to clean. I mean, that car. Yumi was certain the car was "totaled." Yigal quietly bought deodorants, cleaners, and rags. He got whatever he needed, and he cleaned it COMPLETELY. The car was like knew. And Yumi woke up in the morning to this wonderful surprise.

You know, most wouldn't even know where to begin with that, and *[slapping the table]:* he just did it! He told us he was now ready as a man to get married. He had taken care of his parents in a time of need and fear. I mean, it was really a disgusting job. But for him, it was…a gift, mm-hmm. The gift of the right of passage!

## *Angels Lead the Way*

Later, when I had a chance to see what friends had done, I could just feel myself being carried once again. My dear friend Louise had organized everything down to the smallest detail—a healing bear, food, letters, hearts and…that whole condo said, "An Invitation to Wholeness," in every way possible.

*She even had a juicer there for you.*

Yeah, and the juicer, EVERYTHING…it was all there. And Rachel, Yigal's fiancé, came and they wanted to do everything possible for us. They prepared meals, entertained us, and treated us with such loving gestures. They rented light-hearted videos—but you know, interestingly enough, I had no attention span. I couldn't watch for too long. Isn't that interesting? I mean, my whole being required so much inner focus. So we would watch for a little bit, and then I would go rest or close my eyes.

They just did everything, and they cooked, and they straightened up the place, and they massaged me, and…they danced! They put music on and danced for me! I mean they just brought so much joy into the environment. And they'd lie on the floor one minute and be frolicking the next. And the beauty was, that I was awed by how centered and balanced they were, because they both knew that "all is well." That's the part that is so amazing. That's why they could dance. They went out and bought me a new nightgown and new sheets. I mean, it was just wonderful.

*As opposed to tiptoeing around because we have a cancer patient here.*

EXACTLY, RIGHT! My mother has cancer, we need to be very quiet. THAT'S RIGHT! That's right. The opposite. They just really rejoiced.

I had no appetite at that time so Rachel did the little choo-choo thing that you do with little children. You know, like with food on the spoon she'd say, *[sing-song]:* "The Little Choo-Choo is coming into the Sta-tion!" you know. And, "The little airplane is coming into the hang-ar!" We'd all laugh. It was so sweet. And that was really the atmosphere.

I also have a wonderful friend in Israel who sent me an invisible healing treatment (Reiki), all the way from there, each day.

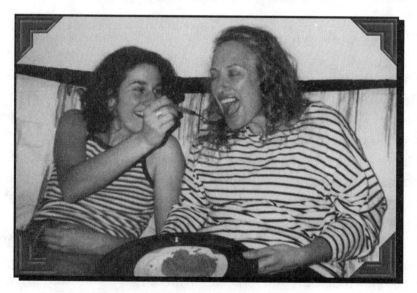

*Rachel playfully feeding Hedy*

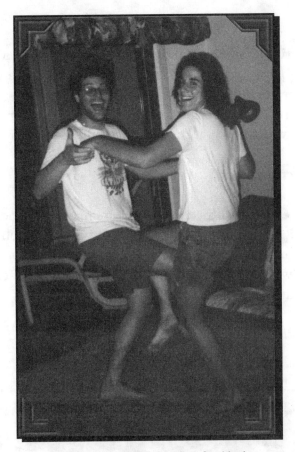

*Yigal and Rachel dancing for Hedy*

From this long distance, she was sending that energy. She told me the precise time she would be sending it. I stretched out on the bed to receive her gift, and I just began to sob. My whole body was shaking. I felt wonderful afterwards.

*Mmmm. I can just picture you spreading your arms wide open and saying, "Here I am."*

She kept doing it, you know, every single day, at that specific time. She said I didn't have to do anything, but just to relax and let it in. So that was another wonderful part of my quick recuperation.

# *And We Have Lift-Off!*

Perfectly timed in this event, was the launch of a rocket at Kennedy Space Center not far from where we were staying. It was the very next day after my treatment. We have a picture of Yumi and I with the rocket going up in the sky over our heads. I was very weak that day. That first day had been a major workout.

*Major inner-aerobics! [laughing]*

Yes! But we went out to watch the launch, and I turned to Yumi, and I said, "You know this whole event is a 'launching.' It's a launching of MAJOR proportion!" He said, "Only you could be feeling so weak, see this launch, and declare for a fact that this whole event is a major launching." He just laughed.

*You're out there all propped-up, and pooped-out...and your spirit is soaring!*

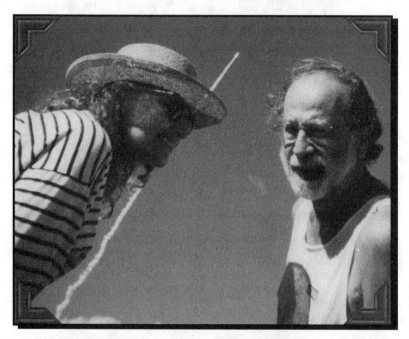

For Hedy, the rocket was a powerful symbol signifying a successful launch in her personal journey.

YES! This was a major launching. I could tell. It was so clear. Here we were, the day after my treatment, standing with others on the beach, in awe of this powerful and successful launch. Such a powerful symbol.

As the Kosher Choreographer would have it, right next to us was a man who had absolutely no hair…a bald, bald man. My hair was still, you know, long and everything. I said to Yumi, "It's not only a major launch; the Kosher Choreographer is also wanting me to see how I will soon look!" *[laughing]* Here was this sweet man, you know, totally bald, and standing next to me, right on cue!

*Another type of "lift-off." [laughter]*

I had heard stories of people who talked about the devastation they felt when their hair fell out. It's interesting because, you know that it's going to fall out, and yet when it does, it's devastating. I knew that my hair was soon going to change, so I decided to welcome the event with a ritual. I thought, how do I embrace the fact that I'm going to lose my hair? The only way I could embrace it is to lose it in a ritual. I decided to lose it purposefully.

So when we returned home, I asked a friend of mine, Ruth, who cuts hair beautifully, to play the role of my beautician in a hair-cutting ceremony. It was so empowering. Several women came for the ceremony, and of course, Yumi was there. And because these women are very connected to ritual, they had written a beautiful blessing for the event. I loved it, because it was a blessing of my whole body. You know how you can get like hair-focused, or cancer-focused. The fact that you had a diagnosis of cancer makes it part of your life, but that's not your life. Well, this is the same thing. You bless the whole body because your hair is part of your body; it's not your whole being. It was a wonderful re-balancing for me.

There is a Jewish hair-cutting ceremony for little boys when they are three years old, and it's called ubscherenish. "Scheren" is to cut. And then ubscherenish is the cutting. And in that

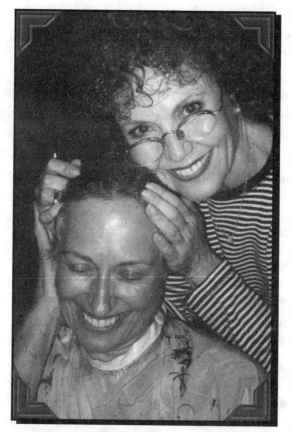

*Hedy during the hair-cutting ritual*

ceremony, everybody who wants to gets to cut a little strand. So the little boy sits there on a big throne, and people come, and they cut a little strand, and cut a little strand, and cut a little strand. So we did that. And Yumi cut the first strand, and I cut another strand, and then everybody cut a strand. And that was like the beginning.

*Your long hair made it possible to have a long ceremony!*

Yes, very long hair. Big hair! And then Yumi gave me a big kiss on my newly unveiled neck. It was starting to show itself at that point. This hair cutting was also a gift for Yumi. He had always adored my neck. I presented my new neck to him!

And, then we did something wonderfully fun. Because Ruth is very talented with her scissors, she was able to give me every hair style I've <u>never</u> had. *[laughing]* Bangs, one side short the other side long, bobbed, layered, short in the back, longer in the front. I mean, it was amazing how she was just creating these hair styles. And while she was doing it, we were talking about hair, skin, pimples, teenagehood, dress, the whole thing about how you look, and the whole evolution into womanhood. We had so much fun. We laughed and joked and cried, and it was truly wonderful. It took about an hour-and-a-half. Then she cut it very short. She cut it like it's now. You know, very, very short. And I wore it that way for a week.

Then a week later, I woke up and saw some of my short hair on the pillow, and I said, "It's time to shave it." So Ruth came back and shaved my head. You saw me that night when you and your wonderful friends came to give me a treatment.

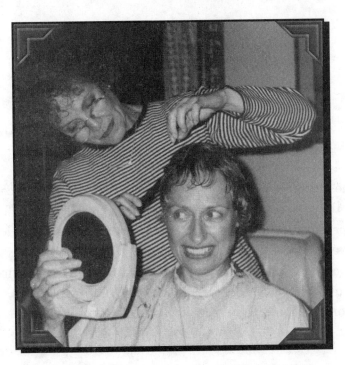

*Ruth gives Hedy one new hair style after another as she trims her hair shorter and shorter.*

*AAAAHHH! That's right. That's right. Proudly sitting in your bed with your newly shaved head.*

There I was with my shaved head. So that was just a marvelous thing. And as a result, I really welcomed my new baldness. I loved my boldness and baldness!

*Also that control.*

Yes.

*You know, you had control over it, it wasn't like just—*

It wasn't happening to me, I was happening to it. I was happenin'. I was happenin'. That really was the thing. And my motto is **I AM HAPPENIN'!**

*AAAHH! [laughter]*

<u>IT</u> ISN'T HAPPENIN'; <u>I</u> AM HAPPENIN'!

*That's a great story. I loved seeing the pictures. Like you say, there's a school girl, there's a girl dating, there's a young one... there's a girl ready for marriage...*

All the girls inside me sort of emerged. And it was so nice to have Yumi there, you know, as a man with all these women. That was very precious. The whole thing was very positive. I still look back and say, "It was very good."

You know, later, I had another "hair raising experience" when I lost my eyebrows. I lost all but three eyebrow hairs on one side. For some reason, they stayed. I named them Charlie, Jeff and Harry.

*The Boys! [Laughter!]*

## <u>It</u> Isn't Happenin'... <u>I</u> Am Happenin'!

*I decided to lose my hair purposefully.*

*I decided to create a ritual to embrace the fact that I was going to lose my hair. It was so empowering... I chose to lose my hair.*

*Consequently, It wasn't happening to me, I was happening to it!*

The steadfast boys that wouldn't fall out. They just hung on, and everything else fell out. That fascinated me. I couldn't help but wonder what made Charlie, Jeff and Harry hold on! *[still laughing]* But one morning, I woke up, and they were gone. I felt bad. I felt very, very bad. I had gotten attached to them. It made me realize a little of what others felt when suddenly their hair fell out. Without warning, my dear friends Charlie, Jeff and Harry were suddenly gone. I was even more thankful that we had had the hair-cutting ritual. I had some control in doing it my way!

## "Bold, Bald and Beautiful!"
### Getting to Know Me, Getting to Like Me,
### Getting to Feel Free and <u>Fuzzy</u>!

*(Once again, Hedy returns and we have more "spatula time.")*

*Today I just want to call in the angels of light, love and healing... the angels that celebrate all that we are, and add to all of this. I ask that, as we speak from our hearts, we experience a blessed and rich time together...and that this time together expands our joy and clarity and inspiration.*

*Hedy, what would you like to add?*

Amen! *[laughing]* Oh, I like it. Oooh, I like it!

Well, here I am, feeling bold, bald—and beautiful, thanks to Yumi! As I said, Yumi thinks I look like an Italian model with my bald head. He sees me with my sunglasses on, my shoulder wrap flying in the breeze, bold and bald and tells me I look like an Italian model! He calls me the "Dalai Mama!" You know, I have no eyebrows, no eyelashes…and much to my surprise, I have even lost all my pubic hair! Who ever thought that <u>that's</u> what they meant when they said I'd lose "all" of my hair! I suddenly look like a little girl. Yumi is even delighted with that. There's just nothing about me that that man doesn't love, and that is so helpful. He looks at me in my bald head, and he loves it. He touches my head, and he loves it. He sees me naked with my newly unveiled vagina, and he loves it.

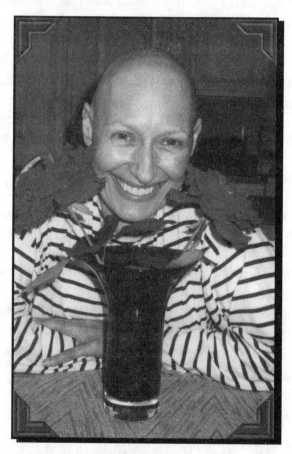

*Bold and bald*

You know what I did? For a while there, I didn't really get acquainted with this new look I now had in my most private area. And I said to Yumi, "You know what? Let me get acquainted with it, **with you**. Help me to see it through your eyes, because you are so thrilled with the way it looks. Help me get acquainted with it." And so we took some time to get acquainted with it through his enthusiasm. Isn't that beautiful?

*It's perfect. It's perfect.*

I was getting reacquainted with myself as a bald woman, (bald in the head and bald down below), through the eyes of a man who is so thrilled with how I look, and who I am, and what I am. He's just with me for every step in this journey. What a gift. I just am so grateful for the way he has responded to every change.

## *"Get Well" Cards*
## *or*
## *"Get Dis-Empowered" Cards?*

What's interesting about getting people's attention after a frightening diagnosis is that, by the time I had stepped into how I was going to do this and was in love with the process, I was also getting cards of condolences. Somehow, I even got one from some organization that said, "In Memoriam!"

*Whoa!*

Cards were pouring in bearing notes of grief and pain. Sweet friends struggled to find words to express how badly they felt and how sorry they were about it all. But, by then I was just thrilled with this next adventure in my life. Clearly, if it was in my path, then this was the one to embrace. My father used to say, quoting the Jewish Talmud, "Who is the happy man? The one who chooses <u>what is</u>."—"The one who chooses what is!" So by then I had chosen what is! And, you know, I was getting these cards that were so sorry about "what is." By then, I had chosen it. It was mine. I was in it completely, "doing it" with every bit of me. Every fiber of my being was now involved in this journey, which is my life. And there was such contrast between people's grief, and where I was at.

Friends wrote that they were "sorry about my illness," but I wasn't feeling ill. They're "so sad about my sickness," but I didn't feel sick. Uh, "what a dreadful disease," but, I didn't think I had a dreadful disease. Uh, none of it fit. Some cards are marvelous and uplifting, but this type of card was extremely draining. They would speak to me through their own wounds, or through their projections of their own fear and pain. They wanted to share what they went through under similar circumstances. Ohh! But the bottom line is that people's intentions were wonderful, and I really learned to translate it and say, all they're saying is that "I love you," and "I'm thinking about you."

*Exactly. A journey like this seems to require a "translator" as your constant companion!*

Absolutely. So, as I received get well cards, I quickly determined that I would only keep the uplifting and empowering ones...even though I knew all were sent with good intentions. The "good intentions" I could resonate to...words of pain, suffering and worry had no place in my life. I quickly decided to file the "good intentions in my heart, and toss the card that contained words that I couldn't resonate to! Eventually, I even found them funny, but I still tossed the card!

*Now that's a sign of fabulous progress. It didn't even get a rise out of you. It just got a laugh. Wow!*

I came to the conclusion that greeting card companies need some pointers on creating empowering and uplifting cards.

*Absolutely. I've noticed that a lot.*

### *Keep the Good Intention, Toss the Card!*

*So, as I received get well cards, I quickly determined
that I would only keep the uplifting ones...
even though I knew all were sent with good intentions.
The "good intentions" I could resonate to...
words of pain, suffering and worry had no place in my life.
I quickly decided to file the good intentions
in my heart, and toss the card! Eventually,
I even found them funny, but I still tossed the card!*

In the meantime, toss—keep—and laugh, toss—keep—and laugh—and translate!

*There you go! Whatever works!*
*You know, wouldn't it be marvelous if somewhere courses were offered in the "Language of Well-being"? You know, the language we were born knowing—our first language? It should be offered in high school and adult education classes.*

That would be fabulous. The Language of Well-being—hopefully a required refresher course for us all.
You know, I taught a training session last week for therapists. There was a woman there whose husband died of cancer many, many years ago. And, even though she heard the news of my diagnosis, she was never able to reach out to me.

*That's all right. If she would have sent you a get well card, you probably would have just tossed her card! [laughing]*

Exactly. She wasn't really ready to connect. She came to the training, feeling bad that she hadn't contacted me. And, during the training, it finally hit her. When I spoke of the "joy of the journey," all she could remember was the end, where the journey with her husband was not joyful. She had forgotten all the joyful moments they had, all along the way. When she thought of me, it reminded her of the END with her husband and, therefore, she couldn't call on me. And, she said now she's remembering the joyful moments with her husband. <u>Now</u> she wishes she had called me so she would have been reminded that there is joy, even in this journey! Uh, still for her, you know, you die of cancer... so at the end, when she hugged me she said, "I'm so glad you didn't die, I'm so glad you didn't die." Well... I'm glad I didn't die, too, but YOU KNOW, WE'RE ALL GOING TO DIE. Whenever, whatever the cause, each of us will die. Mine might be after a diagnosis of cancer, or it might be a quiet, natural transition without anything particular causing it. Who knows? But that's not the point. The point is, it's not that she needs to be glad I didn't die, she needs to <u>be glad for how well I'm living</u>. How fabulously alive I am!

## *Aliveness!*

*It's not that she needs to be glad I didn't die,
she needs to be glad about how well I'm living.
I think a lot of people are sending
me cards thinking,
"OOOOH, she might die," instead of,
"She's more fully alive than she ever was!"*

*Oh! Yes.*

And that's the point she can't quite get yet. And really, I think a lot of people sent me cards thinking, "OOOOH, she might die," instead of, "She's more fully alive than she ever was." I received a wonderful card with a message that I'll never forget. It said, "Hedy you are about to enter a very powerful sisterhood! But... Oy, the initiation!"

# An "Eastern" View

After all these western doctors, last week I went to a Chinese woman that friends were absolutely raving about. She diagnoses you through your ear, using a probe. First of all, let me tell you about these amazing little things in my ear. Do you see these things in my ear?

*Yes, I do...what are they?*

They are seeds...seeds! They stimulate little acupressure points.

My friend has a friend who had advanced ovarian and uterine cancer. And after probing her ear this woman said, "You have another 'tumah' *[mimicking the accent]* in there, there's a tumor, there's a tumor in there." And, of course, she went back to her doctors who had felt sure they had removed everything. She was reevaluated; they opened her up, and, indeed, there it was.

And so Yumi and I went. And what was wonderful about the visit, was that she was going through my ear, and she says, "Brain, oh, Gooawd; heart, gooawd; spleen, gooawd; kidney, gooawd; blood, gooawd." And then she went around my ear, and she says, *[high pitched, sing-song]:* "No cancer, no cancer anywhere." You know, I've known it, but it's kind of nice, you know, to have her just go over my ear and say "no cancer" anywhere.

*It certainly is.*

Anyway, then she said to me, "But you don't sleep well." And you know I hadn't been sleeping well. I've spent many sleepless nights. And she says, "Your body is not digesting the nutrients, so you are weak, you don't feel energetic." And of course that's true. So she's put some things in my ears for sleep. And the first night after she put them in, I really did have a deep sleep. And my energy level yesterday was amazing. I shopped all afternoon with my little daughter-in-law who's visiting from Israel. And we found this store that had everything on sale...so it was even more fun. Everything was just magical. I'm going back to see her on Monday. I'm also having acupuncture periodically. I think both types of treatment will accelerate my recovery.

# Chapter 12

# *Freedom to Soar*

## *The Expanded "Me"...*

The "thing" is this. You know, I decided it would be smart to take a temporary leave of absence from my work and totally focus on health. Yumi and I decided that the office would send a letter of explanation to all my clients. I'd have my office manager take a crack at writing the letter; and, of course, I would massage her letter into the final draft. Yumi handled it for me—but something in the communication between Yumi and my office manager got mixed up. She simply wrote the letter and sent it! And, she selected which clients it would be sent to. Written, signed and sent...just like that! *[pounding the table]:* Boom! *[softly]:* I mean, I have this deep connection with my clients, and this was a form letter! It contained a business-like tone...not the way I wanted to tell them about my absence.

Well, Judie, this hit me in the deepest part of myself. I began to cry; I couldn't stop crying. I was angry. I felt powerless. I felt helpless to do anything about it. It's gone, it's out there. I felt embarrassed, I felt mad at myself for having disconnected so much with my work that my office thinks that they can send letters from me, signed by me, without me seeing them. *[louder and louder]:* I felt sad that the people were going to get this letter and think, "My God, she makes no connection with me anymore? She not only tells me she's not going to be there, but 'she's' not even in her letter? She's not even there! This doesn't even sound like her." *[whispering]:* I mean, Judie, it was—I couldn't stop crying, I couldn't stop being upset. And Yumi had had a hard day, and he couldn't really hold me in my upset. (That one we worked out later. Thank God, we have the skills to do that.) But for a while there, it was tough because I was alone with it. He couldn't hold me. My son and daughter-in-law were echoing sympathetic words in my anguish, "Oh, oh, oh..." as the tears streamed from my eyes, but they were obviously overwhelmed by this "woman who came undone." There's a wonderful expression in Hebrew. Instead of saying something like it's quarter to eleven, they say "it's quarter to cuckoo," cuckoo, like "It's quarter to being totally undone." And isn't that a wonderful expression?

*I love that. I just love that.*

I was "Quarter to cuckoo!" Earlier, my little 3-month-old granddaughter Tobila had a "quarter to cuckoo" moment and now I was taking my turn at a "quarter to cuckoo!" moment. I was absolutely undone!

### "Quarter to Cuckoo!"

*There's a wonderful Hebrew expression...
instead of saying something like
"It's quarter to eleven,"
they say: "It's quarter to cuckoo!"
meaning it's quarter to being totally undone.
And I had truly come undone!*

*Earlier, my little three-month-old granddaughter Tobila
had a "quarter to cuckoo" moment...and now I was
taking my turn! I was absolutely undone!*

So, I called a friend—one who consults with me once a month and is also a friend. And I said, you must have gotten this letter.

And she said, "I did, and I didn't think it was so terrible." And I said, "This is a lot of reality testing for me because I am truly undone about it." She said, "Well, you know, I thought, hey, your office sent it." And then she said something you would love. She said, "Listen, you're taking this leave of absence so that you stop thinking about others. So stop thinking about them. They got the letter, they got the letter."

*She's a very smart woman.*

"Yes," I said to her, "You are very smart." She said, "I learned it from you." *[laughing]* I said, " I'm very glad that I taught you that!"

*[laughing]: There you are...it comes full circle!*

She said, "Here you are, spending all of this time and emotional energy right now, really thinking about this list of people." And it was true. "Now," she said, "I suggest you just let it go." I thanked her and hung up.

Then I thought about writing a letter, a Band-Aid letter... "Sorry about the letter that you received, dah, dah, dah." It was clear that was not to be done.

*It didn't feel good, did it?*

No, it was wrong. No Band-aids. You know, I haven't been in touch with my clients because this whole thing has happened so fast, and, as you know, I've really just gone with it. I am such a one-task person. I've just been totally focused in this other direction. And so this is the first thing they have received. I knew I needed to let it go, but I just couldn't manage to do it. I slowly but surely, slipped into a black hole about everything that I could worry about. I was definitely wand-challenged.

It seemed to precipitate a chain of other unresolved issues. I thought of my unresolved issues with my sister and wondered how this would ever work out? My son Avi and his wife, Sharon, were in a place where things were a little tough for them. Oh boy, that was in there, too. And, Yumi, what's going to happen with his business? In my mind, I could hear the Chinese lady saying, "Heart, GOOAWD; spleen, GOOAWD; emotions, SHOT!" *[laughing]*

I just dug deeper in the black hole. Later in the night, Yumi was wonderful. He really was able to hold my distress for me. You know, he would wake up and he would sort of let me snuggle in and say, *[child-like]:* "I'm just a little girl, and I need help." And he said, "I'm right here." Which is so wonderful that he knows that there is that little person inside that truly needs help. And I said, *[in baby-talk]:* "Say that everything is going to be all right." He said, "Everything is going to be all right." I said, "Say you're going to make it all right." He said, "I'll make it all right." I said, "Say you'll do it with the help of God and all our ancestors." *[laughing]* It was in the middle of the night, and he just said whatever I requested. It was adorable, and it was just what I needed.

When I awoke this morning, I realized that this whole experience has given me an enormous gift. I saw that this scenario, and a lot of my present journey, was about control—and more specifically, letting go of control. It was requiring me to let go of my previous identity. The letter felt as if it colored my clients' perceptions of me. I had to let go of that. Then there was my hair! *[laughing]* My hair, you know, the look that I had to just say goodbye to, because this is the look I have now. The look. The mystique. Everything that I have built up and protected without even realizing it. I mean, I didn't know I was protecting it. When I had to let go of my hair, you know, I thought, "My gosh! This is an enormous thing." Well, the office was another thing that I thought I controlled. I had the illusion that I totally controlled how my office works, and my clients, and what they get and what they don't get.

*How you were represented.*

How I was represented. And now it's shot! It looks like this! *[wadding up paper]:* And then there was the e-mail that went out about me which I had no control as to what was, and wasn't said. It went out constantly, you know, "she burped," "she hiccuped," "she ate some breakfast"...you know, and it's like oooh. Well, it's out there. One woman called me from Washington, D.C. and asked, "Given that you have had a diagnosis of breast cancer and that you have taken Phen-fen for weight loss—do you think that the cancer might have come from the Phen-fen?" *[laughing]* I have never taken Phen-fen! There it is. Judie, it's out there. There's a whole group of people who think Hedy took Phen-fen, and that the cancer must have come from the Phen-fen. It's like, all right. I mean, people will tell stories about you, and think whatever they're going to think.

*[softly]:* Well, when I woke up this morning, I thought, "The beauty of this thing is that I don't have to invest any further energy in keeping up any image. It's blown." *[laughter]* My image is blown. *[laughing]* Yumi said, "They did a blow-job on your image!" Then he added, "Actually, the image of your image is blown!" He was absolutely right!

*[uproarious laughter]*

## The Image of My Image is Blown!

*Well, when I woke up this morning,*
*I thought, "The beauty of this thing is*
*that I don't have to invest any further energy*
*in keeping up any image. It's blown." [laughter]*

*Yumi said, "They did a blow-job on your image!"*
*Then he added,*
*"Actually, the image of your image, is blown!"*
*He was absolutely right!*
*So the beauty is that I can just relax.*

Well, I know that the real essence of me can never be touched, but the image or the identity, you know, the stuff you hold onto that you attempt to protect, is blown. Admittedly, it is silly to spend any energy on protecting that anyway, but I did. So the beauty is that I can just relax.

Part of me knows that. The other part of me is still not too happy about any of it. I want you to read the letter that was sent and tell me what you think.

*[after reading it]: You're right. It doesn't have "you" in it.*

Yes, exactly. You know, I'm very close to these people. It's like me, getting a letter like this from you. Think about it. If I got a letter like this from you, I would wonder what happened there?

*I do see your point, but this is not that bad of a letter. It doesn't take a rocket scientist to see that it's a form letter. My hunch is that your clients are more concerned for your well-being, and less concerned about the fact that it doesn't sound like you wrote it.*

The other thing was that a record wasn't made of who the letters were sent to, so it's impossible to send a follow-up letter.

*Good. You're out of business. How perfect!*

That's right.

*Well, then we can really relax now, can't we!*

Isn't that something.

*I want to emphasize some very interesting points as your story was unfolding. When you said that once you headed for the black hole, you then dragged in "a chain of other unresolved issues"... "everything that you had left in a shaky place." Isn't that interesting how it's all connected? The worse it gets, the worse it gets!*

A black hole.

*You can see how you actually joined the problem energetically with your focus of "Look at what has happened." "This is just outrageous." There you are a wavin' that stick end of the wand. The more you focus on it, the bigger it gets. The good news is that you are sensitive to the discomfort it brought, and tenacious about seeking a better-feeling spot. You vigorously looked for a way to reconnect with your Core Energy. You called your friend for another perspective. She helped you to feel lighter about it, and that got the momentum going in a positive direction. It's like, one thought that's even a little bit soothing, is hooked to another that feels a little better, and so on. It's like a siphon, pulling better and better thoughts to you, and pulling you back out of the hole. Then you slipped and fell in again as your focus returned to the problem. But this time you solicited Yumi to comfort you in the night. It's important to keep doing whatever works to bring you relief. But, first you have to be sensitive to the fact that you're not feeling good, and come to the decision that you want to feel better. You must remember on some level that, "Nothing is more important than that I feel good!"*

Absolutely.

*This second piece is a priceless perspective, and so perfect for times we feel helpless about a situation. That is, whether we are feeling the pain of a "regrettable launch" (something sent off in the mail), or passionately wish we could "suck words back in" which were spoken in an off-moment…it's never the end of the story. Author Deepak Chopra has described us all as moving around in a huge pot of "air soup" and touching each other with our thoughts. Whether we do it intentionally, or not, it's happening. I've come to know that we can enhance anything and anyone, right from where we are. Whether you're sitting in your kitchen, or snuggled between the percale sheets at night, you, as a fully-connected person (tapped into your spiritual source), can make an enormous difference. You can send a package much more powerful than anything written or spoken. In a little over a minute, you can launch a powerful energetic gift.*

Who would guess that you could do so much, in such a tiny amount of time.

*I know. This technique was originally shared years ago by my friend Esther Hicks.[1] It's extraordinarily simple and effective. It utilizes the power of focused thought in this "air soup" we're in. The idea is to hold a pure thought for merely 68 seconds without introducing a contradicting thought or emotion.*

Why 68 seconds?

*I'm told that it's like the boiling point of water. In terms of the time it takes to energetically launch something into being, we only need 68 seconds of pure, focused thought. Actually, just 17 seconds of pure thought is the length of time it takes to attract another thought like it but of a higher, purer vibration. It's like that upward spiral again. The next 17 seconds attracts an even higher vibration, etc. At 68 seconds, you're done! All I can say is, try it for yourself. I think you'll see as I have that it's a powerful technique and ideal for times you feel helpless. Not to mention fun! I've found it so effective that I simply count on the fact that it's a done deal when I finish. In other words, many times it's an issue in which I'm not in a position to determine the success of my efforts immediately. At those times, I still know that I've potentially enhanced the situation and that my gift arrived. You know, I just "know!"*

That's marvelous!

*It goes like this. During the 68 seconds, you merely send good thoughts, or good visions. The important part is the pureness in your focus. It helps to keep it very simple. For example, you might*

*repeat the message that 'All is well.' All of those letters that were
inadvertently mailed and the e-mail messages that you had no
control over were nothing compared to what you can send in this
manner. It's a form of e-mail without a computer. We are partici-
pating in this manner every single day whether we know it or not.
But, knowing you can intentionally send a positive, energetic gift
is priceless in itself. In your situation, it means you can touch
your entire clientele with the love that you are. Just hold a
positive thought for them, without doubting or contradicting it,
and in 68 seconds, you have a launch! And, THIS is mail that
definitely has "you" energetically present in it.*

That's fabulous.

*This technique is perfect for "regrets." It's a wonderful way to go
into "rewind" energetically. Not only does it put you back in touch
with your Authentic Self, but it reaches whoever you are focusing
on, as well. You can even choose to embrace a little scenario. For
example, during the 68 seconds, you might picture your clients as
they read the letter that was sent. Imagine hearing them say
things like, "I wonder what this is all about? It looks like a form
letter. My guess is that Hedy really got overloaded with her
commitments. She works so hard and cares so much. She's probably off in Israel, and her secretary handled this in her absence.
Knowing Hedy, I know she would have written personally, if it
had been at all possible. I have a feeling that she needed a rest.
I'm thrilled that she's taking good care of herself. I'll find out
what the scoop is the next time we meet. In the meantime, I wish
her the best." With just those thoughts of a positive scenario, you
have a very successful, loving launch.*

Right. Right. That feels much better! My office manager really
did it to protect me. She just didn't want me to be bothered with
anything while I'm going through all this.

*Sure. See, you're already massaging this event from a positive perspective. In her case, you might say, "I know she had my best intentions at heart, and she would never do anything to undermine me. And, as she composed the letter, she probably thought that briefer is better—and that she just wanted to take this off my hands." And as you feel that for 68 seconds, you've moved into a better spot about it, and launched a quality gift. The test comes when you can think of her and the letter, and follow with "Ahhhhh. It's all okay. All is well." The tell-tale knee-jerk is gone. There's a saying that others "hear your music, not your words." The music of your soul is loud and clear in this kind of an offering.*

*Admittedly, this technique requires a bit of trust that what I've described is actually happening. I encourage people to just give it a try—especially for those areas when nothing has worked anyway. For example, a relationship that has gone sour. Drop all agendas that you've assumed in an attempt to "fix" it, and just offer a loving 68-second gift each day. Perhaps choose the simple message for them to "remember who they are" (to remember their spiritual connection). The person you're focusing on has total free will to respond or not respond in a favorable manner. You can't force them into connection, but there's a very good chance that you can inspire them into connection with 68 seconds of the "music" from your heart. Everyone wants to feel better when things are uncomfortable. It doesn't feel good to be at odds with others.*

*I have the advantage of having used this technique thousands of times and relate an abundance of miracles directly to this process. I also receive sporadic calls from those who have had amazing success as well—usually they're babbling on my answering machine something to the effect of "you'll never believe this, but..." Oh, but I'm just the one who WOULD believe it! I say, try it. At the most, you're out 68 seconds of your time, and you felt wonderful in every one of those seconds!*

Mm-hmm. I just love it.

*Another priceless benefit of this simple technique is in the area of forgiveness. It's important to forgive others not so that they will*

*feel better, but so that we will feel better. Going back to resentment
and hate being at the stick end of the wand... we need to forgive
others so that we can reclaim our natural position at the star
end. Since you can't be in both places at once, this pure focus
equates to forgiveness. You might look at it as "speed forgiveness,"
or "speed healing!"*

## Beyond Words!

*Others "hear your music,
not your words!"*

I love that... "speed forgiving!" Usually, we're looking at the
person and the outrageous thing they've done and trying to
somehow "forgive that"! In this case, you skip right past all that
and focus on who they really are—or who they'd be if they were
tapped into their Core Energy.

*Exactly. Someday you'll look back on this incident between you
and your office manager and see that it was nothing, and, that
there's nothing to forgive. Poof!*

It already feels that way. It seemed so big at the time, it really
did. And yet, it had an absolute perfection. Oh, Judie. How many
minutes do you spend a day now on this kind of a focus?

*It varies according to how many situations and persons I am
inspired to touch in this way. I include it as part of a whole
routine I do each morning. When I wake up I stay in bed and do
an energetic balancing of my chakras² (energy centers). It's like
an invisible tune-up. This part never fails to entertain Carl.
There I am with my eyes closed and both hands sending energy
to this chakra and that chakra! It's my version of taking care*

*of me before I reach out to help anyone else. (The analogy I've previously mentioned of this being like on airplanes when they instruct you to "put your own oxygen mask on before assisting those around you.") I also set my intention for the day which is always that "nothing is more important than that I feel good," or that "I keep my valve open to my spiritual well-being." Then I move to the floor of the family room to do a stretching routine.*

*Once that is done, I go to the computer to do the 68-second energetic gifts. I find it easier to practice this in writing because writing requires more of a concentrated focus. This part can take five to ten minutes or more. It just depends. I begin with a list of people and situations I want to uplift or enhance, or subjects I personally want to feel better about. In every case, the process not only offers benefits for others but also benefits me. I'm taking care of me. It's such a quick and profound process. It's also perfect for in the middle of the night when I find myself awake for no apparent reason. On those occasions, I don't use the computer. I stay right in bed, send 68-second energetic gifts, and drift back to sleep. It's just a matter of remembering to do it. Once my morning routine is complete, I'm off on my morning walk to practice "feeling good as I walk and pick up litter!" I forgot to mention that I also get dressed!*

Smart woman!

*Later, I'll practice a sort of "spiritual aerobics" as I watch the news or see first-hand dramas in my day. On a normal day, I check out that stick end of the wand for brief periods and then slide right into Home-plate at the star end. Even when I'm touring the stick end, I always know that it's temporary; I know where I'm headed and I know what will get me there. That's a huge "knowing"! Back and forth, back and forth. It's radical aliveness in motion.*

Amazing. What a powerful way to begin each day. This 68-second technique gives me a whole new arena to play in; it's so perfect for times when it's impossible to "do" anything. Those helpless times or moments when life seems to be "on hold." It's the difference between being fully alive, rather than numbed by life. How priceless!

*I know you and Yumi have been very active with a group designed to enhance peace in the middle east. This 68-second technique also sheds a whole new light to what you can do without even leaving your home, without even getting out of bed, and without getting on the plane to Israel. [laughing]*

Yeah. Yeah, yeah, yeah!

*The 68-second technique is merely another way to sniff-out the Kosher Choreographer amidst the chaos. You've already been doing that in one form or another throughout your journey as you found things to celebrate each day, watched for what inspired you, listened to guidance, and then gravitated to what felt right for you. Instead of waiting for the dust to clear and better times to come, you looked for and found God right in your "now."*

That's very true.

*Remember when you were telling me about your friend who was also diagnosed with cancer, and who said how much she hated "the wait"...waiting to get through chemo, waiting to get through radiation, waiting to get well, waiting to get on with her life. But there was no "waiting to get on with life" for you. You celebrated every possible thing in your NOW. You've been relentless about seeking spiritual aliveness (the star end of the wand) in every experience.*

Yes!

*But, back to this letter that was sent and your recent dance with a diagnosis of cancer, I have a hunch that you are somehow*

## Why "Wait!"

*Your dear friend remarked about
how much she hated "the wait" during
her own experience with cancer...
waiting to get through chemo,
waiting to get through radiation, waiting to get well,
waiting to get on with her life..."*

*But there was no
"waiting to get on with life" for you.
You celebrated every possible thing in your
NOW.*

*grooming yourself for a whole new venture, from a slightly new perspective. Something new is coming. And the newness involves you letting go of form, even "form-letters"...[laughter] ...and even your hair and your image!*

[laughing] Yeah, that's such a wonderful thought! Oh, wow. What a powerful vision.

*I have to say that "control" has also been one of my ongoing issues in life. I release control and then gradually take it up again, over and over. We may want to form a group called "Recovering Controllers" or "Controllers Anonymous"! What I keep learning again and again is that our perception in life is truly the only thing we ever have control over.*

It really is. Wow. This one was big. You know, what I'm glad about really is that I gave myself permission to really feel what I was feeling. I sobbed, I mean, SOBBED about this. My little daughter-in-law was holding my hand. And she was putting my head on her shoulder, and she didn't know what to do for me, you know. I was just sobbing, and I was saying, "What do I do? What do I do?" and I guess what I do is I send energetic mail! I get into a good spot emotionally and then launch these wonderful gifts. *It's very liberating, isn't it? You've regained your balance by merely shifting your perception. Your office manager was perfect! She delivered the gift you needed, the priceless gift of letting go of control and especially letting go of controlling your image.*

Right, right. That's so true. Exactly. *[reflecting]:* That's so true. She's perfect. What a gift.

*You wanted her representing you, and she did.*

Absolutely. You know, this technique reminds me of this course that I took years ago in which they did this thing where you dis-create something and then deliberately create what you want. And, I mean, it has that feel to it, but it's just not as complicated. I love this version!

*Another thing that I've found very effective at those times is to ask myself the question: "What's another way I can look at this?" It's the perfect question when you don't have a clue as to what the solution could be. That question has always moved me into better thoughts. It seems to be magical. It's just like Christ said, "Turn the other cheek," or find another way you can look at it.*

Yes! Yes! That's just beautiful!

---

### *Jesus Christ said... "Turn the Other Cheek!"*

*Any time we're stuck in pain or confusion, it's time for the magical question: "What's another way I can look at this?" In other words, turn the other cheek and look in another direction. It leads us to the perfect answer!*

# "Prayer 101"
## *There's prayer...and then there's Prayer!*

You know, after my first dose of (chemo) therapy, I was upstairs resting one afternoon. My energy was very low. Our friends Martha and Jack came over to help where they could. Jack is a wonderful healer and wanted to give me a Reiki treatment. I eagerly agreed.

He began to send healing energy through his hands, working above my body in the most loving manner. But soon Jack began adding prayerful statements as well. He said something like, "Oh, God, cast out this sickness in Hedy." It was so funny the way he solemnly poured out all this heavy, heavy stuff...along with his love for me.

*Mm-hmm, quite a contrast—dark and heavy paired with light and love. Cookies! (see Chapter 2)*

Exactly. Cookies! He had such deep concern about the darkness that he perceived had invaded my body. And I'm on my bed, and I have my eyes closed, and he's doing this prayer as he stands over me. It was just a compilation of words I didn't resonate to; it wasn't in my language. I had my eyes closed, and I must have had a little smile on my face.

I remembered what you had taught me about re-stating (translating) life in a way that aligns you with spiritual connection. I said to myself, "God, what he really means is 'help me relax into the wellness that is natural to me.'"

Then he said something like, "God, please rid Hedy of this darkness."

I said silently, "God, what he really means is, 'expand the light that I am!'" I mean, I really am discovering that I have the power to translate messages into ways that truly serve my best interest, right in the moment! I thought, "Whoa...I am turning this around, right NOW!" It was just as simple as that. I was able to accept his wonderful gift and yet align perfectly with my truth. I just translated it into another language. Although I knew it was coming from love and an intention to embrace me, we really were speaking two different languages!

*How perfect. Translating into the language of Well-being. As more and more people acquaint themselves with this language, translation will be less and less necessary. It will be a wonderful moment when you can immediately embrace the same language and soar together! In the meantime, the translating serves as an instantaneous re-connector and keeps you moving in the direction you want to go.*

His language is actually the more common one. It's a fine language; it's just not the one I speak. But, it's so wonderful to have people speak your own language. I mean, when your letter came, it was in my language. It was just so wonderful. There was nothing there I had to translate. But very few people speak this language. You call it the language of Well-being, and I think it's a perfect name for it. I'm not denying anything, I just speak another language. I resonate to the language of Well-being.

*And the lighter version helps your immune system; the heavy, dark language stifles it, unless you are able to transcend it. Your translation of Jack's prayer was a great example of praying from an open valve...affirming what already exists. It's about our alignment with our true nature, and asking assistance in opening us to receive what's already ours. Take light, for example. As my friend Esther says, "There is light...and the absence of light, but there is no darkness—there is no 'dark switch' on the wall. There is only the absence of light." We've merely let in less light, or turned down our rheostat with negative thinking or even negative praying when we're trying to get rid of something (stick end of the wand). So, you might say that we have health...and the absence of health (absence of the stream of Life Force or stream of well-being), rather than disease.*

That's a great way to put it.

*So even when you're praying, pray for what you are wanting rather than what you are trying to eliminate. Even if you don't know what it is you want, you usually know how you'd like to feel. Articulate that: "I want to expand my feeling of clarity, knowingness, flexibility, freedom, joy, a peaceful heart, love, passion for life, appreciation, steadiness, strength, aliveness, and spiritual connection. Heavenly Father, open my heart, my mind and my body to allow the well-being that is natural to me. I know that your light continually flows through me and lights up every cell in my body. Please help me each day to acknowledge your ongoing, unceasing Holy Presence in all that I am."*

Ooooh, Amen! What a beautiful prayer. What an open valve!

*In other words, "Lighten up!"*

Exactly.

*It's so easy to become consumed by frightening lab reports, odd sensations going on in our bodies, doctor appointments, medical or surgical treatments, physical discomforts and the like. Most people would lump it all into an unpleasant dose of reality. But what we declare as "reality" is merely our <u>perception</u> of what's going on in life. (You may want to read that again!) The fun part in all of this is that we always have a choice as to how we perceive life. Always. We can control our perception of life. Isn't that fun?*

Fun and powerful. It's exactly what my mother did in the German prison camp. She chose to see it differently and to see the prison guards differently. Consequently, miracles happened.

*Yeah. That's a perfect example. Many of the things we experience feel so much bigger than us. I love an advertisement that is on one of those blood pressure machines at our supermarket. It has a picture of a man who appears full of joy and in radiant health. The caption reads, "I am stronger than diabetes!" Then it talks about how he has made the choice to take excellent care of himself (star end of the wand) even with a diagnosis of diabetes. It's about remembering who you really are, beyond the scary data and bodily symptoms, and choosing to make that bigger. It's the BIG YOU that you want to take into that doctor's office for your next appointment. Just like when you insisted on getting centered before going in for "the news" of the diagnosis that awaited you.*

There's such a big difference in the experience.

*Another simple but very powerful way to do it is to rehearse it in your mind ahead of time. Even write it out like a script in a play. Something like, "Today, I'm going in for a breast biopsy. I want to find things to appreciate all along the way. I want to enjoy all interactions with each member of the staff who will be caring for me, and feel nurtured throughout the experience. I want to feel my spiritual and emotional well-being throughout the day. I'm going to watch for every possible way to feel good throughout this experience, because I know the priceless gift that it provides for me on all levels. I choose to take the spiritually-aligned 'Big Me' in for this appointment today. Here We go!"*

That's it! Here "We" go! It's the only combination to have.

*Absolutely. And for those who choose to tough it out alone, there's never a shortage of stories about how outrageously unfair their lives are. There's never a shortage of persons who are experiencing an absolute flood of overwhelming events in their lives. From their perspective, it's just "happening to them" out of the blue. It's rotten luck. It's the way the cookie crumbles. It's the pits. But it's actually a prime example of that old giant Poker Game in life I was referring to earlier. (see Chapter 10) Some call it the Law of Attraction. It's a big perspective. It seems even bigger when you're the one in a lot of pain. To think that you had anything to do in orchestrating these gut wrenching experiences for yourself, seems absolutely absurd. Some people are ready for this perspective and some are not. Are you?*

*Regardless of how you think this happened in your life, it can easily precipitate an all-time low in even the best of us. But, hang on! There's good news in reaching that lowly point. It's actually a priceless moment when you are most apt to shout a powerful prayer. Yes, if you're lucky, you'll fall into a heap and shout emphatically, "I—give—up!" It's a powerful, pivoting moment. It's shouting a prayer of your new declaration in life. It's also the moment when God says, "Good! Now 'We' can begin." (In other words, now that you've stopped trying to bang things into place, stopped pushing against what you don't want, stopped whining, begging, bargaining, and pleading. . . now you and God can begin once again!) In effect, you've suddenly removed the blindfold from your eyes, the ear plugs from your ears, the spiritual straight-jacket from your body, opened your clenched fists, and reconnected with your true nature. In that instant, you took your*

## *I Give Up!*
### *(What a powerful prayer!)*

*That "all-time low" is a priceless moment*
*when you are most apt to shout a powerful prayer,*
*"I—give—up!" It's the moment when God says,*
*"Good! Now 'We' can begin."*
*(Now that you've stopped trying to bang things into place,*
*stopped pushing against what you don't want, stopped*
*whining, begging, bargaining, and pleading...*
*now 'We' can begin!) In effect, you've suddenly removed*
*the blindfold from your eyes, the ear plugs from your*
*ears, the spiritual straight-jacket from your body, opened*
*your clenched fists, and reconnected with your true*
*nature. You "let go, and let God." God had never left.*
*You merely freed-up what was there all along,*
*the Light of God.*

*attention off the negative drama and relaxed. You "let go, and let God." God had never left. You merely freed-up what was there all along, the Light of God. Now that's a powerful prayer!*

Wow. You know, you hear stories of that happening all the time. They sank to what for them was their lowest point in life, and it suddenly turned around for them. Things immediately began to get better.

*Yes. Shouting a prayer of "I—give—up!" instantly has you sporting huge, divine, catcher's mitts on each hand You are now back in the ball game. God steps in as a "relief pitcher," pitching a new game. The fun thing is that this game of "relief" can be played while lying flat on your back, totally relaxed (or even limp), with catcher's mitts resting in a palm-up position, ready to receive all good that is yours. You've shouted your prayer. You're breathing more deeply with each breath. You lie there in this totally non-resistant state, willing to receive good things in your life. As time progresses, you notice that life begins to work—doors open, the right people show up, the perfect person suddenly calls, you feel lighter, and synchronicity is sprinkled in each day. Life is flowing in every cell. It's time to shout another powerful prayer that's one of gratitude. You shout, "Thank You! Thank You! Thank You!" That is fabulous praying, and it's a fabulous new alignment.*

Or as you called it…"speed healing!" Gratitude is so important.

*Yes, it's the simple paired with profound. I love it. We always make things so complicated. Think about prayer with regard to the analogy of the magic wand. God is at the star end of the wand. A prayer to eradicate pain and darkness is only effective to the extent that it stimulates you to slide to the star end. In other words, if thinking of casting out darkness stimulates you to focus on the light, you've made it to the star end. But that's the long route! And, for whatever length of time you're busy trying to cast out the darkness, you stay at the stick end. So, ask yourself as you pray: Are you praying to embrace what it would feel like to have what you desire... or praying to get rid of the problem? Are you affirming your good, or pushing away the bad? Is your prayer one of disconnection, or connection? God always answers us, but it's only in a connected state that we can receive.*

Yes! Who wants all that meaningless sliding around on that stick... sliding that may or may not lead to the star end? I want that rich exchange from the beginning. The first is just delaying the second. A prayer of connection... now, <u>that's</u> prayer!

*Amen!*

## Prayer versus The Pray-er

*So, ask yourself as you pray:*
*Are you praying to embrace what it*
*would feel like to have what you desire...*
*or praying to get rid of the problem?*
*Are you affirming your good,*
*or pushing away the bad?*
*Is your prayer one of connection, or disconnection?*
*God always answers us, but it's only in*
*a connected state that we can receive.*

# Chapter 13

# What's the Real Message?

## The Message in the Massage for the "Cancer Patient"

I got a call from my gynecologist's office. Her receptionist said that there's a woman whose mother's life was touched by cancer, who wants to give a gift to people whose lives are also touched by cancer. She does this by paying for a massage. She remains anonymous and the person who receives it is anonymous. And I thought, wow, that is just beautiful. And the woman said, "Yes, we do this for our patients with cancer." I said, "Oh, I am not a patient with cancer." She said, "Oh?" I said, "I had a diagnosis of cancer, but I don't have cancer." And she said, "Oh, yes, I understand, I understand completely." And she continued to talk, but soon was using the expression "cancer patient" once more. She gave me a number to call, and instructed me to ask for the "anonymous massage for cancer patients." And I said, "Oh, but I just want to repeat again, I am not a cancer patient." And she said, "Oh, yes, oh yes, of course, I understand. Anyway," she said, "when you're ready, just call us." And I said, "Okay. This is a wonderful gesture."

This morning guidance said, "Don't go. Pass the gift on." I didn't try to figure it out. I just called and said, "I want you to know that I am very touched by the gift, but I want to pass it on." I said, "I have lots of friends who do massage, and I'm very well covered in that area, and I just want to give it to someone who actually needs it more, and so I'm passing it on. Thank you so much for the wonderful gesture." And I put the phone down. I said to my son and daughter-in-law, who were sitting there, "You know, even calling someone a 'cancer survivor' always pulls them back to that." I said, "When you get married, you don't say you are a 'survivor of singledom,' you know. Or childhood, I'm a 'childhood survivor.' You just say, 'I grew up!'"

Then, when you referred to me earlier as being "recently diagnosed with perfect health," I realized that the only people I want touching me are those who are aligned with that. I don't want to be massaged by someone who has the perception that they are "massaging a cancer patient" or a "cancer survivor." It just won't do. And it was just so clear as I was lying there on your table today, and as you were touching me with your "nuclear heat" and your inner knowing that I am in perfect health, that that's really the only way I want to be touched. Yumi touches me that way. I realized, that because I had to say it twice to this woman, that it wouldn't be understood. It just wouldn't, and I would be receiving the gift as a cancer patient. That's not for me.

*No, that's not you. Of course, you're the one with the spiffy new identity, anyway! [laughing] You're right. The therapist would be*

## Touching the Divine in Others

*And when you referred to me as being*
*"recently diagnosed with perfect health,"*
*I realized that the only people I allow*
*to touch me are those who know that.*
*A massage as a cancer patient won't do for me.*
*I am not a cancer patient. And it was just so clear as*
*I was lying there and as you were touching me*
*from that place of my perfect health,*
*that that's really the only way I want to be touched.*

## The Language of Well-Being!

*I said, "You know, even calling someone a
'cancer survivor' always pulls them back to that."
I said, "You know, when you get married,
you don't say you are a 'survivor of singledom.'
Or for childhood, I'm a 'childhood survivor.'
You just say, 'I grew up!'"*

*doing therapy "on a cancer patient." You're not a match to that.
What a wonderful gift it would be to offer a "wellness massage"
to celebrate life! That would be such a wonderful message silently
paired with the massage.*

That's such a beautiful thought. You know, on my last appointment for (chemo) therapy, there was a brand new sign that said:

> "Welcome cancer survivors!
> From the time of its
> discovery and for the
> balance of your life,
> an individual with cancer,
> is a survivor!"

I asked the woman at the desk if she saw anything wrong with that sign. She looked at it, checking it for spelling, etc. It didn't occur to her that there was anything wrong with the term "cancer survivor!" Who wants to be a "cancer survivor" for the rest of your life! I'll admit that it's wonderful to survive and to be alive. But I feel that it does us a disservice to continue to hold that title after the fact. I want to be a "thrive-er" and one who embraces life, health, wholeness, balance, and aliveness!

*Yes! You know, perhaps the sign could instead read something like this:*

# *Just for You!*

*We include a blessing, just for you, at no extra charge!*

*We bless your eyes, that you may see God in all things.*

*We bless your ears, that you may easily hear the whispers of His angels.*

*We bless your Spirit, that you may remain strong and connected to the "You" of you.*

*We bless your body, that you may fully love it.*

*We bless your clear knowing of the unceasing, unseen, cellular miracles that are normal within your body!*

*We bless your perception, that you may perceive life in a way that serves you well.*

*We bless your ability to remain focused on what you are wanting more of and what you will say "Yes!" to.*

*We bless your sensitivity to how you are feeling in each moment, your inner guidance system, that allows you to feel your way into spiritual connection.*

*We bless your knowing that "Nothing is more important than that you feel good" in any moment, for it is then that all things are possible.*

*We bless your willingness to steadily find things to appreciate, and to practice an attitude of gratitude on a daily basis.*

*We bless your ever-expanding ability to laugh and "lighten up!"*

*We bless the Authentic You!*

*We could give each person a magic wand to take with them!*

What a difference! Now, that's what I resonate to! '

*Me, too. The sign you first read reminded me of that silly vision I've mentioned before of running towards "the light" with a long stream of toilet paper stuck to one foot. Terms like "cancer patient" or "cancer survivor" just represent more toilet paper.*

*Chapter 14*

# The Incessant Demand for Radical Aliveness

## The Emancipation of a Green Napkin

Oh gosh, this is such a good story. We went out with friends for the first time on Memorial Day. Many places were closed for the holiday, so we went to the gorgeous Sebring Country Club in Orlando. And you know, it is such a fabulous place. It wasn't so long ago that Jews were not allowed into places like that. Here I am going into the Sebring Country Club, bold and bald! Well, you know, bald heads chill easily and it wasn't long before my head got cold. The green cloth napkin at my place setting provided the perfect answer. I made an instant hat, a dooda hat, which is a thing with three knots—one on my forehead, two on the sides.

*[laughing] A "dooda hat!" Did the green match anything that you were wearing?*

Not particularly! I was wearing this wonderful black and silver thing, with this green dooda hat!

Soon, I told our friends about the havoc this journey had played with my image. The dooda hat made that even funnier. Then Yumi topped it off by chiming in with his favorite line, "Every image deserves a good blow-job!"

*Blow-job! [laughter]*

But we talked about how friends surface with a preconceived "image" of a person who's "diagnosed with cancer." With that image in mind, they call and speak in a "poor you" tone saying, "When can I come to visit you?" We're mismatched. They're over there focusing on sickness, and I'm over here—having a good time. We don't fit. We laughed about what the perfect answer might be that would sort of shock them into the realization that perfect health is what we are enjoying here, one that would teach them a new role to play in all this. Yumi said *[playfully]*: that I should say, "Sure, come and visit. I charge $160 an hour." Or I should say, "Sure, what's on your mind?" (as if THEY must be calling with a personal problem), or I should say, "Come when I'm closer to death." *[laughing]* Or I should tell them that "Celebration is daily here," or "If you come, come to enjoy the fun. Align with that." Some sort of gentle answer that aligns with what I'm about, takes into consideration people's intention and generosity, but teaches them a more appropriate role to play in my journey. Align with my radiance and friendship, not a diagnosis! Another image to blow—the one of the sick, or dying friend. We're getting really good at these blow-jobs! The dooda hat was perfection.

## *The Power of Boredom!*
### *(Heads-Up Cancer! You're Powerless Here!)*

I sat up in bed in the middle of the night last night and had a huge realization. It was the following: I am **bored** with cancer! I just am really bored—bored with the subject. I've also found that this "being bored" is very empowering. It's like it has no more excitement than molasses. Whenever I honor that, I have a lot of energy. *(There's your cue! You're at the star end of the wand!)* And when I don't honor that, it sucks my energy. *(There's another cue, stick end!)* It is just phenomenal. It's so clear that cancer, and fighting cancer, is at the stick end of the wand. I'll give you an example because it was very powerful.

Some friends came to see the little office that we have, to see if they want to rent it for their practice. One of them said, "Well, Hedy, how are you and what's happening?" And I said, "Oh, you're not going to believe this. I am so bored with the whole thing." Well, they absolutely burst out laughing. And after that, the one friend was telling me something about her career, and why she's looking for a room, and it's because there are so many horrible dynamics going on where she works and—then she stopped and looked at me and she says, "You know what, I'm bored with it, and I'm not even going to tell you about it. We're just going to talk about the possibilities for my life."

And we began to laugh. And I said, "You see, isn't that interesting. If you kept digging in the stuff, you're there—but if you say 'enough of this thing,' you're immediately over here, creating life." And the two of us were mutually thrilled with the whole thing. She said, "Thank you so much." I thought I'd tell her about magic wands on another visit!

On another occasion, Yumi and I were enjoying a snack with friends in our living room before dinner. One of them said, "And so, Hedy, what's new with your cancer?" And I said, "I'm so bored with that whole thing." She looked at me and said, "Of course." And we just moved on. Which was like brilliant. I mean, I'm telling you this "bored with it" is brilliant!

*It's empowering.*

Absolutely, empowering. You know, last week I decided to take Louise out to dinner in celebration of my perfect health. And the beauty of the event was that I picked her up at her house at 7:00 p.m., and we proceeded to drive through an outrageous rainstorm.

*Oh, I know. It was wild here as well.*

There were lightning strikes in every direction, and the rain came down in sheets. And when we arrived at the Alfe's restaurant, it had changed to this gentle, lovely rain. We saw several skies on our trip: the "blue sky" and "the sun-still-out sky" when we began our drive, then the sun a little lower with the clouds increasing, then very dark clouds in the pouring rain, followed by a very bright red sky. You know how it looks after the rain; it's just so beautiful. I mean it was suddenly brilliant green, lush, alive, sparkling, enriched and big. The whole place was perfection. Louise and I thought about what a phenomenal gift this was to see nature perform so dramatically all around us, and arrive perfectly fine, with enhanced beauty everywhere as a result…as if Mother Nature had spiffed up just for us.

*We might want to tell her not to be so vigorous next time!*

Yes, yes. But at the same time, it was very symbolic…a storm, coming out on the other side in a gentle rain. And then sitting, of course, at the best table in the house right over the lake, a view that was ever changing, ever perfect, ever magnificent. It was just phenomenal. It was just like I felt…sparkling and magnificent, after being vigorously spiffed up inside and out!

*You're right. What a great symbol of your recent journey.*

And Louise and I were talking. But instead of heeding my own inner direction (which is that I am bored with this thing), I talk about it. And it's amazing how it sucks my energy dry. It wasn't until this morning that it became clear to me that I spoke from an image-building point of view to aggrandize myself. I heard myself telling Louise, "Oh, I think that God has given this to me because I had to face death, so that I can really speak from a powerful knowing." It was very powerful sounding, very convincing. Even I was very convinced as I listened to myself. "Oh, I think God gave this to me,"—isn't that a phenomenal statement?—"so I could let go of my image, and not really care what people think, and really not have fear." And this morning

I thought, *[in a low guttural voice]:* "Bullshit, **bullshit, bull-shit!"** I don't know why I got this, but I got this. I got rid of it, and I'm living. It's like, who in the heck cares? *[laughter]* You know? But you can really get on the soapbox with it and create a whole big drama about the thing. And this morning I woke up with a sense of, "Hedy, this is such bullshit. Just shut up, and do your life!"

*[softly]: Yeah, oh yeah!*

You know..."shut up!" I mean, who cares. But it really drained my energy. I could feel it while I was talking. I could feel that it was just *sliding* me to the other side of the wand, rather than focusing on the beautiful ever-changing sky over the lake. We did that, too. I mean, we did talk about other things, but that little piece right there was very draining. And, it became so clear to me that with some people in my life, I could be so easily seduced into that spiel. Rather than saying, "You know what, I'm so bored with this," and let it go and just move on. I'm learning. Just realizing this morning that piece of the conversation was bullshit, was enormous for me. Because you know what? I could have people absolutely spellbound over that type of presentation. They unwittingly want to hear about my journey from that perspective. Oh, my God!

*Profound, and seductive.*

They'd be saying, "This woman is PROFOUND!"

*And bald. [laughing]*

And bald! "Oh gosh, we must listen to her. She really knows about this." I now know that "that" sucks my energy dry. And "that" is over; it's the past! Here is where I am. "That" isn't for me. That's very profound. It was the voice of my inner guidance loud and clear saying, "That's bullshit!"

## *Here is Where I Am!*

*But instead of heeding my own direction,
which is that I am bored with this thing, I did talk
about it. And it's amazing how it sucks my energy.
And I talked about it, but I realized this morning, that I
spoke from an image-building point of view to
aggrandize myself. And this morning I thought,
[in a low guttural voice]: "Bullshit, **bullshit, bullshit!"**
I don't know why I got this, but I got this, and it's over.
Here is where I am.*

*What a gift. Finding cancer boring means that it has no "emotional clout" with you. It's powerless, and you're empowered. The diagnosis of cancer is neutralized with your feeling that it's boring, and you instantly slide to the star end of the wand! Wheeeee! Your energy soars!*

It did. Yes, what a gift. This "I'm bored with it" is a powerful gift indeed.

# A Support Group: Supporting the Solution or the Problem?

## *What's in a Name?*
## *(Plenty!)*

*Recently I was with my best friend, Pat, in Virginia, and visiting her mother who was in the hospital. While on the hospital elevator, we saw a sign that said, "Come to the Living With Cancer Support Group." We both looked at each other and gasped. Who would want to focus on "living with cancer"? Now, we both clearly knew what they meant and how good it feels to be so thoroughly understood by those who have had a similar journey. How nice to help ease the experience for each other. But it would serve them better to come at it from another angle. How about "Choosing Radical Aliveness!...A focus group for anyone who is cellularly-challenged!"*

*I know that many attribute their strength and well-being to the experience that their support group provided for them. It feels so good to be understood by those who have also walked in your "cellularly-challenged shoes." It's great to receive practical suggestions and new strategies that ease life on so many levels. Being able to express your fears, concerns and frustrations to others who really know what you're going through, admittedly feels wonderful. Each of those benefits, when properly used, birth the "empowered us." You might think of them as providing a lift; a boat ride from the Land of Challenge to the Land of Well-being where we reclaim our power. Once at their destination, the occupants eagerly disembark onto the Land of Well-being, ready to begin again with new goals and seeing things in a new light. They have a renewed sense of "aliveness." Now that's a boat ride! Perhaps that's even a luxury cruise!*

*Unfortunately, there are the other boat rides in which the occupants are so busy telling and re-telling their story, that they forget to disembark! Week after week, they regurgitate their fears, frustrations and difficulties as they "share" with others.*

It's like gathering others to lend a compassionate ear. But there's more to "supporting aliveness" than a compassionate ear! You must take it further.

*Precisely. You can tell how well any group is serving you if you check with your emotional guidance system. What does it feel like to experience the sharing. When it's over, are you feeling as if your spirit is thriving? Is there a renewed sense of aliveness? In simpler terms, do you feel good? Do you feel empowered? If so, that's for you.*

*Beyond the sharing, wouldn't it serve everyone well to meet with the purpose of celebrating life and expanding the creative ways that life could be embraced more fully? (even with physical limitations) Wouldn't it serve everyone well to choose a name for the group that also massages a perception of aliveness, like the laryngectomy group who called themselves The Chatter Boxes! Now, there's a name!*

Yes, Yes!

## What's in a Name? (Plenty!)

*On the hospital elevator we read a sign that said, "Come to the Living With Cancer Support Group." Who would want to focus on living with cancer? How about "Choosing Radical Aliveness!... A focus group for anyone who's cellularly-challenged." Or, how about the laryngectomy group that called themselves The Chatter Boxes!*

*Hedy, if you were to create a support group that supports health and wellness, what comes to your mind?*

It would definitely be one in which we would express our aliveness. For example, aliveness expressed through movement of some kind. In the past, I have created dance groups for the purpose of free expression. I must dance. Unless I dance, I'm not expressing a huge piece of myself. I've made a commitment—I must dance once a week. A support group that includes dancing would tap everyone into their aliveness. Each person would naturally participate to whatever extent is possible. If their bodies aren't able to move, they can dance in their minds. Whatever the form, we would all close our eyes and move to the music. Movement is a must.

*They just do whatever comes natural to them during the music?*

Yes. We start by really warming up through music, so there's a whole routine I put together in various rhythms to warm-up the whole body. And when we're done with that, I have various pieces to it; one is free expression with incredible music playing. Everybody just moves to the music in whatever way feels right, at that moment. Another way I've done it is to pair off in partners and "mirror each other." That, too, is just a profound thing in movement. And then some creative routines done on the floor in free expression. Other routines done in circles, as we touch each other. It's a whole routine that is fantastic. It's freeing, expressive, wild, soft, tender, and outrageous. It's very important to me to express myself without words. You can't bullshit through movement. So it is a very important piece in my own life.

But back to your original question. I feel that any support group should have a focus of expressing aliveness.

*And spiritual connection!*

Absolutely, a valve-opening experience. Imagine finding all kinds of creative ways to express aliveness. Most only know of the other kind of support groups where they bare their soul, and share their triumphs and fears **about cancer**. Oh, God, sharing, sharing.

*Sharing of pain. You know, there's sharing, and then there's* <u>sharing</u>*! Perhaps some guidelines could be set to keep the disempowering stories (for the one listening and the one telling it) to a minimum. People tend to want to drag it all out, blow-by-blow. The most important part is for human spirits to soar. Perhaps stories of that nature could be sandwiched between experiences promoting aliveness, so that everyone begins and ends with uplifting, life-promoting thoughts, even for those terminally ill. The idea is to be very alive right up to the moment of rebirth on the other side.*

*Author Carolyn Myss has coined the term "woundology."[1] That's the style of expressing in which you reach out to others in an attempt to see where you've suffered similar hurts and challenges in life. You bond through the pain you have in common. You speak woundology. Wouldn't it be better to bond through aliveness instead of pain? Bond with someone who helped your spirit soar?*

Absolutely!

*What if the format was one in which you came to enhance, celebrate, mirror, and magnify you at your very best, on all levels? A format that chose avenues of:*

- *singing,*
- *dancing,*
- *art,*
- *sharing energy (sending love through your hands),*
- *sharing magnificent dreams,*
- *sharing uplifting visions,*
- *sharing positive gratitude journals,*
- *making magic boxes that are filled with pictures, words and items that connect you with your Authenticity,*
- *guided meditations...guiding you to spiritual connection,*
- *foot massage,*
- *sitting up straighter,*
- *putting on make-up,*
- *smiling,*
- *pairing your name with a power-filled accolade, "I am the Resplendent Ruth," "The Radiant Rosanne," "The Magnificent Marie," etc.,*
- *sharing stories of "aliveness" (in daily life, and after life!),*
- *massaging perceptions,*
- *sharing ways to be "with" others who have since made their transitions, instead of being "without" them. (They've merely changed form.)*

That's such a fabulous list.

*All of those things have the potential to stimulate aliveness. As one woman put it, "Just because I have a diagnosis of cancer, doesn't mean I have to look sick!" She made it a ritual of putting on make-up and wearing something nice each day. So often we think we have to first feel better before considering some options. When actually, those very options are the key to feeling better. Sit up straighter, put on make-up, dress in something pretty (or handsome), and smile. All provide internal and external cues for well-being.*

Yes, that's it.

### Fake It 'til You Make It!

So often we think we have to
first feel better before considering some options.
When actually, those very options
are the key to feeling better.
Sit up straighter, put on make-up,
dress in something pretty (or handsome), and smile.
All provide internal and external cues for well-being.

*It could be an evening of whatever connects everyone with their Authentic Self. A tonic all around!*

Your little Thursday night group is another perfect example of celebrating life.

*It sure is. You know, that's our play group, our place to Spiritually expand and tease out the best in each other. One night, for example, we had each person take a turn standing in the center of the circle and tell the others who they really are, beyond any limitations. We had a magic wand that could grant them any wish. We asked that they fast-forward to "whoever" or "however" they passionately wanted to be, and to "be it now." It was their job to introduce us to this new "them," as if it were already true. They were to tell us what they felt like and what they do while living from that perspective. It was extremely powerful. Those of us in the circle would simultaneously lend our energetic support of that version of themselves. At the end, we'd all sit quietly and silently embrace this vision of them, for a few moments. The power of two or more fully-focused human beings, embracing a common vision is phenomenal.*

It creates miracles. I just loved your Thursday night group.

*Speaking of miracles, I am reminded of the fabulous story Richard Moss tells in his book* The Black Butterfly[2] *about a woman named Laura who was terminally ill with cancer. She was also diabetic, on kidney dialysis, had large tumors, and many health problems. At his workshop, he divided the participants into groups of four; one person in the middle with the other three surrounding them. The three played individual roles of support and inspiration as the one in the center either danced or sang until they became one with the dance or one with the song. Or until the "dance danced them," or the "song sang them" effortlessly. Ultimately, Laura completely reclaimed her health, following her participation in the singing and dancing. She danced for hours and sang for hours while being empowered by the three others. The large tumors totally disappeared. She "forgot about trying to be healed" and "fell into aliveness." She became a person "vibrating at a new note."*

*After months of documenting her perfect health with her physician, she and her husband sold everything, bought an R.V. and began touring the country, celebrating life. Now, that's the style that I resonate to!*

Fell into aliveness...How fabulous!

*Richard Moss states, "The singing exercise is a way of teaching prayer. It is consecrated to the aliveness that always awaits us. It is the music of one's own being that becomes the inspiration for the song."... "The singing and dancing exercises demand that we find balance between will and surrender, between trying for more and accepting exactly where we are... To experience the sacrament of the moment, that space where the song sings us, where life lives us, we must be willing to let go and keep letting go... In a sense, we are having a love affair with life."*[3]

That's just so fabulous!

*Along with the singing and dancing exercises, he also orchestrates another exercise in which the group enters into energy sharing, focusing their energy on Laura. She perceived it as a healing ritual, acknowledging her wholeness,*[4] *not as an attempt to "fix her." Just to celebrate the truth.*

Yes! Yes!

## *Laura's Story*

*The participants were instructed to dance until the dance "dances you," or sing until you become one with the song. Laura "forgot about trying to be healed" and "fell into aliveness." She became a person vibrating at a new note.*

*As I've said before, even the word "healing" denotes something that needs to be healed or fixed. I find it more empowering to call it a celebration of wellness in which you hold a space for the person to acknowledge their wholeness. You don't try to deny disease; you merely focus on seeing them whole and fully alive. We've grown so used to certain terms that are actually hindering, rather than helping. We've heard them so long that they sound normal!*

Absolutely.

*Whenever I give a treatment, healing energy is flowing from my hands while my mind is embracing the best version of "them" that I can envision. For example, a man in his late 30's came to me with a terrible back problem a couple years ago. He hobbled from his car to my massage table in a great deal of distress. In using the analogy of the wand, his pain and dysfunction were at the stick end and total relief was at the star end of the wand. In order to assist him, I needed to do it from the star end. I had to conjure a vision of him at his very best and hold that focus for him. I knew that total relief would mean that he felt strong and flexible, and that he moved with comfort and ease. So the entire time I was flowing energy to his back, I was enjoying an ongoing vision of him as a skilled ballet dancer. I saw him looking flexible and strong, and he moved to the music, dancing the ballet. Then I pictured him moving easily and gracefully while doing Tai Chi[5]—again celebrating the truth of his back—that it was strong, and flexible and comfortable. I mentally joined his magnificence. When he left about an hour and a half later, he was in total comfort.*

That's fabulous!

*I didn't try to "fix" his back; I merely provided an energetic touch-stone so that he realigned with his healthy, perfect back. I hung out at the star end of the wand, while silently, energetically entic-ing him to join me! You might say it was a support group of two physical people and a host of invisible angels. A mighty fine group! Anyway, it's a great example of the amazing influence of focused thought.*

That's the kind of support I'd want! How profound. You know recently an acquaintance left a message asking me if I'd like to join with others, including her daughter in a "cancer support group." I told Yumi that if she had said, "Hedy, I know some phenomenal people who are going to be in a support group to celebrate perfect health and life and aliveness. And they are phenomenal; one's an artist, one's a writer, one's my wonderful daughter...would you, who are so incredibly fully-alive, be part of it?" I would think, "This sounds amazing! I'd like to see what that's all about."

This week I received a call asking whether I'd speak to a "Cancer Survivor Group" in October. I said, "Sure I would. I just don't know whether they will appreciate my point of view, because I would want to tell them what I've learned, my experience, and how the term 'cancer survivor' is just an absolute no-no." You don't call a person a "survivor" to begin with, because that means like, my God, they might have died. Who cares? What took over is life, not death! Let's call it what it is. Let's call this what took over, rather than what didn't happen. How unfair to keep bringing them back to "that close call with cancer."

*And, how many other groups are doing the same thing, whether it be incest, rape, uh-*

I thought exactly of that. They say things like, "I am an incest survivor!"

*I have a neighbor who said, "I am a rape victim survivor." That was ten years ago. She's still trying to hold a space for it.*

You got it. *[laughing]* That's right.

*I thought of saying, "First of all, I'd change that label you've given yourself." Wooh!*

It means that every single day, you go back to the incest or rape, instead of realizing you are alive and well. In doing so, you resist the very thing you want—peace and well-being. But, most people just don't know any other way, and it has become normal to express it like that. But that "cancer survivor" thing made me think of all sorts of statements of this kind that I had never thought about before. Like "holocaust survivor"—FORGET IT! Let it go! But, many go back there, and back there, and back there. So "there" is where they "are." They're missing a huge chunk of "here and now!"

*How well put! You know, Steven Spielberg has created a project[6] that assists holocaust survivors in recording their story on video. Many of the people coming forward have carried the painful memories with them for years and years and yet have never spoken about it to others. On one level, you might say that for years it's been stifling their flow of Life Force. Although the gesture is an attempt to record these stories so that they will be preserved for future generations, I see it as potentially having a very different benefit. It seems to me that by telling your story on tape one final time, it has the potential gift of helping you to let go, knowing that it's recorded for posterity. You no longer have to be the "keeper of the story." I see it as a tremendously healthy way to move on. But, for those who still want to keep remembering, they can choose to play this story again and again. It's a choice.*

Absolutely. Do you know the motto of holocaust survivors is, "Never again!"? Now, think about that. When every day you say, "Never again!" you are there. Instead of spending energy saying "no" to the holocaust, you must instead say "Yes!" to life. It's a big point of view, you know; some are ready for it and some are not.

## *Now __This__ is Doctoring!*

Yesterday we went to see a radiation oncologist that had been recommended by a good friend. He turned out to be a 40-something Scotsman who recently married for the first time. He married the woman who was the nurse that took care of his mother when she was dying. He came into the room and was so obviously in love, and so happy, and just oozing with delight about being alive. He had the cutest big blue eyes. He sat down, and right away it was like "Wow!" He had gone over my records and said, "I'm just missing some of the information. What about progesterone and testosterone?" We gave him that information. He said, "Look at this (pointing to some of the reports). All of this is so good." I said, "You've given me good grades." He said, "Oh, well, you are doing all this." Anyway, he asked about the chemotherapy. And I said, "It's 4 times C-A." He said, "That's the best. And how are you doing with it?" And I said, "I'm doing very well." And he says, "Oh, I am so pleased to hear it." And he was just a delight, a DELIGHT! Anyway, he was called out of the room several times and each time he said, "I'm so sorry I have to leave," and "So sorry I have to…" I said to him, "We've set aside the entire morning to meet with you, so just do your thing." So we sat there and he was in and out.

Well, then he started telling us about his marriage. I said, "I understand you've just come back from your honeymoon." "Oh, yes." And he told us about his honeymoon, and he blushed about the romantic things. And I said, "You know, you're talking to the right people. We teach couples how to have an alive and conscious relationship!" He replied, "You do? One of these days I hope you'll sit with me and tell me all about what it is you're doing." (All this with that wonderful Scottish lilt, you know.) And *[whispering]:* a doctor who spends time with you on life, as he shares his delight about his marriage, his honeymoon, his excitement. Not, you know, with his nose buried inside your record. It's like he was saying, "We'll talk about <u>life</u>, and we'll also do 'this'! I mean, after all, you've come for 'this,' but—"

*Yeah, we'll throw "that" in too.*

We'll throw that in. Isn't that gorgeous? Isn't that just gorgeous? I mean he's such a mensch. And I said to him, "Do you know Dr. Walker?" (You know, my beloved surgeon there at Ellis Clinic.)

He said, "No, I know of him." And I said, "You've got to know him, you know. Robert Walker is a mensch, and you are a mensch. You two really have to meet and get to know each other."

So we made this phenomenal connection with him. He was a nuclear physicist, and then decided to also become a doctor. He's also a computer nerd. Yumi noticed that he had this little computer in his pocket. He pulled it out, and spent half an hour showing Yumi all the little buttons. They're really bonded now! Two physicists, in heaven with a computer.

You see, that's doctoring because it's medical excellence paired with life, it's blending the scientific with the human being. We'll have this consultation and, yes, we'll also throw in the computer demonstration! Well, of course, as a physicist he understands radiation in a way that is off the charts. And, he talked about being very careful of my lung and heart during the radiation. I could tell he is really going to take every precaution. You know, I felt like he's watching out for my heart, and watching out for my lungs and—you know what I mean?

*He's looking out for your best interest in every area.*

Every area. He's going to make sure that they're really very well protected and all that. I mean, I felt wonderful with him, just wonderful. And so, as we were leaving he said, "Oh, by the way. You had cancer, cancer is in the past. We're just doing a little preventative therapy." Judie, I was in tears. I can't help but wonder if he understood the genius of what he had just said. I'm wondering, is he aware? Is this something he does? He is so innocent. You see what I'm trying to say? He was so pure in spirit and so innocent and spoke straight from his heart. I know it wasn't just a casual remark that he felt he'd "throw in," just so I could be relieved. I could feel the truth in what he said. He said it because he had looked at everything, you know, at all of the pieces, and he said it's in the past. Isn't that lovely?

I said, "Yumi, did you see what that man just did? Is that a doctor or what?" I mean, a doctor in the fullest sense of the word,

## *Real Doctor-ing!*

*He told us exactly what was going to happen,*
*and arranged the appointment at the exact time*
*I wanted it. He did everything possible to*
*acknowledge the human being in the patient!*
*He not only talked about medicine,*
*but he talked about life!*

*You see, that's doctoring*
*because it's medical excellence paired with life.*
*It's blending the scientific with the human being.*

letting this woman know that from everything he's seen, it's over. Cancer is in the past. Judie, up until now, other than the Chinese doctor that I went to for herbs, none of the doctors had spoken those words.

Now, you have known this, I have known this, Yumi has known this, but the western doctors had not been willing to put words to it. The Chinese lady said, "No cancer anywhere." I had purposefully combined the east and the west, the "Ying and the Young" as Yumi calls it. (You know "Ying" is "Young" in Yiddish.) So Yumi says, "It's the Ying and the Young." *[laughing]* It's fabulous hearing the "Ying and the Young" in agreement.

But back to this doctor, I don't think he realizes what he did that day. I don't think he has a sense that he was being a doctor when he shared about his wife and his excitement and how loved he feels. And that he played with Yumi on the computer, and that that had more energy to it than basically just reading the report, which was his job. He told us exactly what was going to happen, and arranged the appointment at the exact time I wanted it. He did everything possible to acknowledge "human being" in the patient!

*Absolutely profound!*

I don't know if he realized, <u>that</u> is real doctoring. I don't think he knows what a healer he is. He'll hear from me about it. I will put it in words for him, so he begins to really know what he does. He's a healer. Like Robert Walker is a healer. And, oh, and then he examined me. Now, you know, a lot of people have palpated my breasts. And I now have categories of breast palpation. *[laughter]* His exam was superb.

# *Pondering Pivotal Moments*

*It's so fun watching this ever-growing list of "pivotal moments" tucked into your conversations with the medical establishment. Your quest to find your Boob Dream Team offered potential growth even for those who would not ultimately be chosen. What fun! You sort of massaged their reality into a new perspective. For example:*

•*The doctor who said, "In the case of <u>your</u> cancer, Mrs. Schleifer..." and you responded with, "Stop right there, Doctor, this is not <u>my</u> cancer." And the doctor who insisted on seeing you in his little examining room—who upon your request to meet in a more suitable area, replied, "Mrs. Schleifer, this is where I see all my patients." You responded, "But, Doctor, I'm not your patient yet. I'm Hedy Schleifer, and I haven't chosen to be a patient yet. I may choose to become one, but I'm not one yet, and I must talk to you as Hedy Schleifer, and I must speak to you as Robert Brown!" (not his real name) He was inspired to spend more time with you and even see you to the door. You ultimately touched his heart and perhaps reminded him who he really is and why he went into this profession.*

•*The woman who wanted to schedule you for a complimentary massage that was routinely offered to all "cancer patients" and you replied, "But I'm not a cancer patient." "Oh, I understand," she said, "You're using positive thinking." At some later point, she may understand the power of massaging from a perspective of the recipient being in radiant health versus massaging a "cancer patient!"*

• *The nurse in the recovery room who offered you a medication to help you calm the shaking you were experiencing, and you told her all you needed was to hold her hand and be allowed to cry. She had never thought of just holding the patient's hand. There has to be a good chance that she's offered to hold the hands of patients that followed.*

*Then others came along. But in this case, they ultimately massaged your empowerment.*

• *Your surgeon, Dr. Robert Walker, whom you recognized as compassionate and on the leading edge. You said when he examined you, it was as if he touched your breast like a prayer. "His touch was sacred."*

Yes, absolutely sacred!

• *The Scotsman, the radiologist who took time to be human and to offer a statement that "Your cancer is in the past. You no longer have cancer. We're just doing a little preventative maintenance." By blending medical excellence with real human-ness, he earned your title of another "real doctor."*

Ummmmmmm.

• *The oncologist at Ellis who showed you a totally supportive style of chemotherapy. It would be administered in an extremely comfortable environment and with family support in mind. As you once told me, "When she examines your breast, she leaves no corner unturned." She gets in there, and you feel as though she has a hundred fingers. Those hundred fingers go into your breast, and you feel like when she is done with you, there's nothing in that breast she hasn't felt. If she says you're o.k., you're O.K.!*

*These brilliant scientists, physicians, nurses, human empowerers would indeed be on your team! You found each of them as you felt their presence, and they felt yours. It was a match.*

Absolutely! My dream team!

On one visit my oncologist said, "You know, you don't have to see Robert Walker when you come back in September, you can just see me." And I said, "I'm seeing both of you! I wouldn't want to miss that prayer over my breast that he does...or the hundred fingers that you examine with either! I've driven all this way for a breast prayer and a hundred investigative fingers." *[laughter]*

*I was telling a friend of mine (whose daughter had a diagnosis of cancer) about your response to the offer of a "complimentary massage for cancer patients." And she said, "Well, if she is not a 'cancer patient,' what does she describe herself as?" And I said, "Well, she's a person who has now been given the diagnosis of perfect health [laughter] and is celebrating life! She doesn't have time for anything that doesn't line up with that!"*

That's exactly right! Exactly right! *[pounding on table]:* A person who was given the diagnosis of perfect health, is celebrating life, and is bored, bored with that conversation of "woundology"! That's it!

## Will the Real Hedy Please Rise?

*I was telling a friend of mine
(whose daughter had a diagnosis of cancer)
about your response to the offer of a
"complimentary massage for cancer patients."
And she said,
"Well, if she is not a 'cancer patient,'
what does she describe herself as?"*

*And I said, "Well, she's a person
who has now been given the diagnosis
of perfect health and is celebrating life.
And she doesn't have time for anything
that doesn't line up with that!*

*And I would add, that you're a person who has been freed from previous perceptions that were hampering your flying. Because of that, Mission Control (or the Kosher Choreographer) has officially granted you a whole new air space.*

Exactly! And this new air space is so freeing. It's really been wonderful.

The other thing I realized is, as I continue to be bored with it all, I will honor that for as long as it lasts. When the next realization emerges, I'll move on. I already have friends who say I will always have this in the back of my mind, the diagnosis of cancer. They say, "You will never not think about it." Bullshit! I'm already not thinking about it. *[laughter]* You know, I'm already not thinking thoughts like "Is it in there? Is it not in there? Is it truly over with?" And if ever in the future there's a diagnosis of something, we'll just go from there. In the meantime, there's only room for good things in my thoughts. Think about the diagnosis? Of course not! Why think about boring things!

*Do you know how many people would purchase that perspective if they could actually buy it? They're going insane with "what if-ing" and "what's that-ing."*

Absolutely. This freedom is exhilarating, and I would wish it for everyone.

## So You Want to Help? Join the Fun!

You know, I've decided to have a week of celebration in every direction. Recently, I got word that our cousins were coming. These are cousins who are devastated by "the news" and dearly want to help. But, I could already feel their heaviness and they hadn't even arrived yet. So I talked to one of them and said, "There's been a change in spirit here." I said, "You had decided you wanted to help, and there is a new way to do that." I said,

"It's to celebrate and have fun, because I'm bored. And because I've just been diagnosed with perfect health." He said, "Great." Then magically, our friend's beach house became available. It's so funny. It's like, as soon as I spoke to him, it became available and it's just gorgeous. So we're going to the beach house, with the cousins. They're bringing all kinds of food and now it's turned into a light-hearted celebration!

Another thing I've done that I think is wonderful, is that I decided to ease up on all the dietary restrictions I imposed on myself in the beginning. You know, low fat, and organic foods, etc. This week, I've blown every restriction. I said, "For one week, I am having fun with food. My appetite is back. I'm just going to go for it." I have, and it's been wonderful, just wonderful.

*What was your favorite?*

My favorite is dessert.

*Really! And what did you choose?*

Mmmmm! I chose something different every night. Last night, it was chocolate soufflé at Alfe's. I mean that is beyond belief. It's this little soufflé that has a marvelous soft crust of chocolate. When you cut into it, there's this dark, gooey, warm chocolate that *[laughter]* oozes out with this vanilla cream all around. The night at the Sebring Country Club, we all shared chocolate mousse pie, and a chocolate and hazelnut delight. And the night before, Yumi gave me vanilla ice cream with kiwi slices and whipped cream. *[laughter]* I just let myself go, you know? Yesterday I even had like candy, disgusting, you know, chewy candy. For about the last two and a half years, I had limited my desserts to just once a week. I think I'll go back to that eventually, because it's a very nice discipline. But for this week, I truly am celebrating. I'm celebrating with food. I'm celebrating with movement. I'm celebrating with singing. I'm celebrating with clothes. You should have seen how I got dressed up Tuesday morning, the day that wonderful doctor said his beautiful words, "You <u>had</u> cancer, it's in the past." I had put on my beautiful white barmitzvah dress—it's a goddess dress, and I added a big necklace that I love to wear with it. Yumi said, "Hedy, are you not overdressed?" I said, "It's Tuesday." He said, "Oh, I forgot, it's Tuesday!" (I'm celebrating anything and everything about Life!)

*You're celebrating TUESDAY! [laughter]*

It's Tuesday! He said, "Oh, I forgot." *[grinning knowingly]*

*I'm celebrating morning. [laughter] I'm celebrating the fall of a leaf! [more laughter]*

Right. It's so marvelous. So, I arrived at the doctor's office all dressed up. I was all dressed up the whole day. I went out that night in that dress, and I said to Yumi, "Look, I mean even if it was just for Tuesday, it would be the perfect dress. But, for a doctor to also express what I have known, that regarding cancer, 'It's in the past.' There's another fabulous thing to get dressed up for!" How many doctors say this about cancer? They don't dare. They don't dare to put data out like that. They're so afraid that there's, ooh, something here or there. Isn't that incredible?

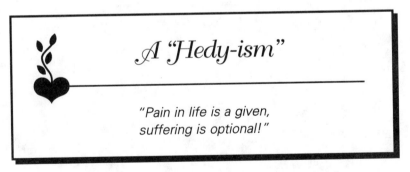

*A "Hedy-ism"*

*"Pain in life is a given, suffering is optional!"*

# $\mathcal{P}$erception is a Choice

## *Third Time's the Charm!*

My experience of the third dose of (chemo) therapy has really been quite incredible. I was much better prepared on all levels. I had a medication to help me to sleep on the drive from Sarasota to Orlando. I had also received help from a Chinese treatment prior to the therapy. Something that made a huge difference on the second and third treatments was the addition of the meditation tape you made for me. I listened to your soothing voice over and over during the therapy. It provided a continual celebration of the magnificence of my body, and a welcoming of this liquid. Welcoming! Who'd ever think you could come to welcome this liquid! I now see the resistance that I had about that first treatment. I really hated the thought of putting chemicals in my body! They were anything but welcome! So I really learned to align myself with the very thing I resisted before. I arrived home without any sort of car sickness or anything. I progressed from major vomiting on that first dose, to feeling weak with slight queasiness after the second dose, and after this third dose, which was the strongest so far (they progressively increase the dosage for each treatment), I've done even better. The stronger it got, the better I've handled it. So, once I completed this shift in perspective and welcomed this liquid, it created an entirely different experience.

*It's just fascinating to contemplate the role alignment plays in your experience AND the role your perception plays in that alignment. It's so freeing to realize that we can control our perception about anything, even something like this. We are free to choose our favorite version. The perception is only helpful to the extent that you feel wonderful about it inside. In other words, that old cliché about "painting black...white" just won't cut it. And just saying the words won't do it. You have to find an angle that you personally resonate to and feel wonderful about. It's different for everyone. The acupuncture treatments, herbs, medications to help you sleep, the meditation tape, all played important roles in that you perceived them to be of help. They were hand-picked by Hedy Schleifer and had you feeling wonderfully aligned.*

They truly did. Your guided meditation simply made me feel fabulous as I relaxed and welcomed this liquid.

Something else that really made a difference between that first treatment and the two that followed, was my decision to take a leave of absence from work. Initially, I thought that I'd divide myself between my work and the therapy. Then I realized that this journey IS my work! I don't plan on "doing cancer" again, so I want to do it well! I am totally focused on the richest possible journey.

*And it's really paying off!*

You know, after each treatment, it's like you're in a "zone" for the first two days. You know, your body—

*Is busy.*

Is busy. "It's busy," what a good way to put it!

*Busy re-establishing balance.*

You've got it. Your body is busy, and you feel it. You know, it's like pregnancy...like the beginning of a pregnancy. Your body is a factory, and now it is doing something with the stuff that's in it. It's like when the egg and the sperm get together—only this is a different kind of marriage of things inside there!

*A rather unusual pregnancy! [laughter]*

And so, the body is very busy. But on Monday, I went back to the Chinese woman. She is such a delight. She really is a healer. Anyway, she put stuff in my ear, and you know, I said to her, "I'm a little queasy." She mirrors in a sympathetic tone, "Oh, queasy." I said, "Yeah, I'm a little nauseous." "Oh, nauseous." I said to her, "You know, I have very little energy." "Little energy, oh." You know, she just mirrors everything you say, and just has this real caring look. She performed acupuncture in a couple of spots and said, "That's for queasy." And then put four more needles in, and also used something that heated the needles called moxy. I call it moxy poxy.

*A "moxa stick," or "moxibustion stick."[1] It reminds me of something we used to light fireworks when I was a kid. You light the end and it sort of smolders and stays hot. As I recall, they use it in acupuncture to warm the needle so that it stimulates energy flow even more.*

Ahh...a moxa stick. Well, her assistant, who is the most beautiful Chinese woman you'd ever want to see, goes around each needle with that moxy thing. Anyway, I came home exhausted. And my body was very busy. But the next day, my energy was steadily increasing like magic. It truly is from inside—it's beautiful to see how energy rises. It rises through the chakras.[2] Isn't that true?

*Listen to you! Yes, it does. It rises through your energy centers.*

It does! It does! It's unbelievable. *[laughter]* I never had experienced this. But now, I've just been watching my body. It rises through the chakras slowly, at a pace that is all its own. It's very touch-ing. It came up and up and up and up, and when it got to the top, I had energy all over! I am flabbergasted with it. *[laughter]*

Tuesday it began to rise, and by Wednesday, you know, on Wednesday night I had that sense of being "just bored with this thing," and had all of my energy back. My stomach was fine. Thursday, Friday and Saturday, I had total energy. Sunday morning I got up and, boom! Low energy. Who knows from what, but low energy. I hadn't slept, but who knows what it was.

*The body was "busy" again. You know, there are many invisible cycles to honor, as your body regains its balance.*

Absolutely. There's a lot of shifting around.

Another example of this busy-ness, is that my blood is doing its own thing. I have to tell you a very funny thing. They took a blood sample and Yumi has asked for a FAX of the report. I never would have, but you know, Yumi's a scientist who loves to see these things. Well, it turns out that the low-normal for blood cells called monocytes is four. I have zero. Now, it could be low, it could even be half a percent. But I have zero! Well, when you take a look at this thing, it's like, whoa... zero! Now that doesn't look good to us. (Valve closed!)

So we put a call in to the nurse. We got a recording. And I left a message, "Hello, this is Hedy, and we just got the blood report and an item on it is really concerning us. Could you give us a call today? I'm home all afternoon." Well, she didn't return my call. I thought, this could actually be a serious thing, but my guess was that if it were serious, they'd have called. You know, they're watching this data, too. That thought made me feel better. (Valve opened!)

So the next day, while we're driving to Miami, Yumi calls again on the car phone. "We must speak to the nurse right now. Please get us through."

And he does it in such a phenomenal way that, of course, she's on the phone. "HELLO, YUMI, I HAVE LEFT A MESSAGE,

AND I HAVE—DAH-DAH-DAH-DAH."

Yumi says, "We are concerned about the monocytes being zero."

She says, "OH, YOU DON'T HAVE TO WORRY ABOUT THAT. THE ONLY THING YOU HAVE TO WORRY ABOUT IS THE GRANULOCYTES. THAT'S THE ONLY THING WE WORRY ABOUT."

Yumi said, "I just want to know what it means. What does it mean to have zero monocytes? It's my wife we're talking about here!"

She says, "WELL, TELL YOU WHAT, YUMI. I WILL TALK TO THE DOCTOR, AND IF THERE'S ANYTHING TO WORRY ABOUT, I'LL CALL YOU BACK." But it didn't give us the peace of mind we were looking for. I mean, the zero is still there.

*There was your "cue." You needed to get your valve opened back up, one way or another!*

Exactly. So we decided to let it go. We thought, I guess if there's anything to worry about, she'll tell us. That felt a little better. And then we pondered that we still don't know what it is, but, I'm alive and well, and I have good energy. I'm able to drive the car now, and all of that. And that thought felt even better.

*That's a perfect example of talking about an offsetting issue with the goal of feeling better about it. It's a fabulous, soothing technique for things like this. That report of your monocytes remained unchanged. But your perception changed. For your body's sake, your mind's sake and your Spirit's sake, "Nothing is more important than that you feel good." The greatest thing you could do for your monocyte count is to feel happy! Suffering (and blaming) is optional!*

Yes! My body was already singing another note. And, because I'd moved toward greater balance, my monocytes had probably already gone from "zero" to "some!"

*Absolutely! We like "some!"*

Admittedly, the delay in their response was an interesting piece in this journey. It's the only piece that isn't quite in place— getting a reasonably prompt response after calling with concerns. I plan to write a letter about availability, and the hotline, and all of that. That's going to be very important for the future people. I've also decided to send a gift of bubble bath and a letter to this nurse. I think she needs to know that people understand her and see the burden she carries, and that taking a bath in this bubble bath every once in awhile will provide a wonderful rejuvenation for her. Yumi and I are going to be sending her lots of love. That's all I'm going to do with this.

*Look at this entire scenario. You witnessed yourself feeling the level of energy rise in your body and became fascinated with the way your full energy returned. When it disappeared for no apparent reason, you were willing to embrace all of the "shifting" that was continually taking place as it returned to balance. The "busyness" was the sign of your body working perfectly. When you found yourself frustrated over the results of your blood work and key medical persons unavailable, you used it as the cue that it was. You chose to find thoughts that felt better, thoughts that bolstered your well-being. You also thought of a loving and proactive plan to bolster the nurse in doing her job, and to improve communication for those coming after you. And finally, you released it! So many people would have fallen into an emotional heap, interpreting this as a sure sign that "something's going wrong," or "I thought I was getting well, but..." Thoughts like, "All is well," and the metaphor of it all being like a "pregnancy" and full of "appropriate busy-ness" wouldn't have entered their minds.*

Yes, yes.

*I think I'll rename you, "Sparkle-Plenty." You shine, Girl...even without monocytes! [laughing]*

Yes, I said to Yumi, "What I can do on zero monocytes is phenomenal!" *[laughing]* Yumi said, "You are a walking exhibit of interesting phenomena!"

## Manicure...Pedicure... Perception-icure

*(Taped June 5, 1997, with one chemotherapy treatment to go.)*

*(Once again we're talking to the spatula.)*

We must do one of your lovely prayers. I love listening to it.

*Yes, yes. Let's just take a nice full breath. Uhmmmm. We eagerly invite our angels of light and love to join us. We call on our "Authentic Selves" to be fully present. We bless in advance all of the words that come forward as we speak from our hearts, and embrace the gifts that life has continued to offer. Amen, Amen.*

Amen! Oh Amen, UH HUH!
    Judie, the main thing I have to say today is that I <u>feel wonderful!</u>

*You look it! There's an absolute glow about you. Your eyes are sparkling, you're wearing lipstick. A flow, and a glow...Life Force must be oozing from every pore. OOZING!*

Yes! *[laughter]* This is great.
    It is so marvelous, it is just so marvelous. I must tell you that yesterday I called to make an appointment for a manicure and a pedicure today. The woman I go to is just marvelous. But, she only had the time for a manicure at 12:00. I said, "If anything opens up that has a two-hour slot, I'd love it." So this morning, the person at 1:00 o'clock *[sing-song]:* ♪♪ "just cancelled" ♪♪ so that I could have the manicure and the pedicure! *[laughter]* It was just marvelous timing. It's been this way throughout my life,

you know…but on this recent journey, it's been accelerated. It seems that, as I open up more to life, it opens up to me.

*Daily synchronicity!*

Exactly. And speaking of synchronicity, while I am having my manicure, five of my friends show up, one by one. Three are really good friends, and two are more "acquaintances." I hadn't seen these friends in a very long time, but they had heard of my diagnosis. And each one of them had a different reaction. One said, "I can't believe you look so good." And I replied, *[melodically]:* "Well, it's because I **am** so good." She said, "What do you mean?" I said, "Well, I am 100% wellness and complete health and—" "But are you doing chemotherapy?" I said, "Yes, I am, as a preventive measure. I have actually learned to welcome it. I've actually learned to have a relationship with it that has grown and grown, since the time I first encountered it. You might say it's a blossoming relationship!"

And the second one said, "Oh, Hedy, I can't wait to tell the community. Everybody is so worried about you. I mean, you are the picture of health, and the picture of well-being, and the picture of radiance, and…" on and on. And she said, "I know you only got this thing so you could teach about it." (Which is what I hear from many people.) She said, "I can already hear you teaching just in what you've said to us."

Then the third friend showed up, and she immediately had this big frown and said in a pathetically sad tone, "Oh, Hedy." (There's a lot of love between us.) I said, *[grinning broadly]:* "Shar-ron, that frown has got to go! It has nothing to do with anything!" And she said, "Really!" And I said, "Yes, you can have a big smile on your face, and just welcome me knowing that all is well." So it was very nice to just connect, you know, the way women do at the hairdresser and with the manicure/pedicure thing, and just reunite.

*"That frown has got to go!" What a wonderful way to put it. The*

*language of Well-being is spoken here!*

Yes, yes. That frown has got to go. I had a manicure and pedicure, and they had their perception massaged...a "perception-icure!"

## Are You in Remission?

You know, I called a cousin the other day and she said, "Are you in remission?" (They just keep wanting me to say I'm in "remission.") And I said, "Oh, no." I said something to the affect that I'm done with it...it's out...it was a diagnosis...they took care of it...I am in perfect health! She says, "Oh, that is so wonderful." And I could see that even for her, this remission thing was a little bit worrisome, because who knows how long the remission will last. She really resonated with my full declaration of well-being.

*You know, for many reasons, the term "remission" is like the first chance people have to breathe more easily; it's a term paired with relief. But while it's certainly better than an active disease, it's also, for many, like waiting for the other shoe to drop. It seems too bold for most to lay claim to their perfect health. Cancer and other diseases often feel like "sneak attacks" that occur when you're taking your health for granted and busy "doing life." Better not tempt the attackee! Better hold on to an ongoing relationship with cancer, out of respect for its power. (Like, better focus on the "stick end of the wand where cancer is, so I can keep an eye on it.")*

That's it! It isn't a full embrace of health and well-being.

*Instead of remission, a more empowering and playful expression might be, "I have transcended the diagnosis!" or "I moved right past remission and on to perfect health." "I have transcended it!"*

Yes! I have transcended it!

# *Are You in Remission?*

*People keep wanting me to say
that I'm in remission!*

*I tell them that I'm done with it...it's out...
it was a diagnosis...they took care of it...
now I'm in perfect health.*

*This remission thing was a little bit worrisome
even for my friend because who knows how long
the remission will last. She really resonated
with my full declaration of well-being.*

*That's right. Now others can really join you in embracing a whole new vision of you! You've enticed them to join you at the star end of the wand.*

*Asking about "remission" is the only way most people know to inquire about promising news in your progress. Anything more seems like too much of a leap. After all, we're talking about cancer here! Who'd think to ask if you're now back in perfect health? Even doctors prefer to speak in terms of remission until a certain number of "cancer-free" years have gone by.*

*The words you choose to declare your perfect health are only words unless they are paired with an inner knowing. You can feel the difference. You know whether you are feeling totally comfortable as you proclaim that you have "transcended it," or whether there's a little doubt there and you're pushing against cancer. But, in any case, it's always a place to start until you grow into the fullness of it. It's obvious that you were totally comfortable with all declarations of your perfect health.*

Yes. Yes.

*As Mahatma Ghandi once said, "Be the change." It's important to find every way to "be it." After months of identifying themselves as being one who's diagnosed with cancer, it's really necessary to develop a strong relationship with their healthy selves. After all, that drama has been so BIG. It's time to make their "healthy self" even BIGGER! They need to have a "getting-to-know-the-healthy-me" agenda each day. Writing in a daily journal is a great way to get to know this new healthy "you" and to grow in "cellular confidence." It's a great way to practice "being the change," and to get comfortable expressing it so that it feels solid when you tell others. For example, if you're writing in a daily journal, you may want to examine aspects of your life by looking through the eyes of one who is in perfect health. Write about what new choices you're making with this renewed confidence in your health—write about that in detail. Live it in advance. Be the change.*

What a powerful statement, "Be the change." It says it all.

*Yeah. It's also good to spend quiet moments talking to your body, praising it, reflecting on its strength and aligning with your internal magnificence. Reflect on the unseen miracles taking place in your body at that precise moment. I know you've just done this intuitively all your life.*

Yes. I must admit I've been fascinated with the way the Kosher Choreographer designed it. I've appreciated it on so many levels.

*The idea is to practice being aligned, and truly fine—instead of trying to convince anyone that you're fine. There's a fine line between "claiming to be in perfect health" and "reclaiming your perfect health." (Valve open!) There can be a bit of a "push against cancer" in the first version. You are the only one who will truly know which side of the line you are on. You'll know when you really feel the truth in it. When you can confidently say things like, "I've transcended the whole diagnosis!" "It's just plain gone!" "I spend my time celebrating life!"—and you feel a true sense of "cellular confidence"—you're really in business! That means you feel wonderful inside.*

Yes. It's like celebrating life from a place inside me that is totally free!

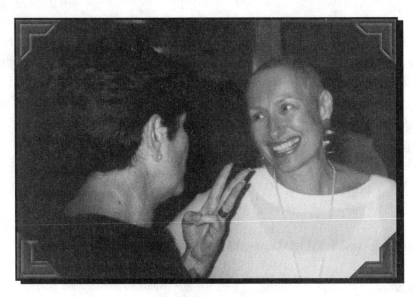

*Hedy, totally free*

# *A Feather Amidst the Rocks!*

*You know, Hedy, I've always known you to be so positive, joyful and light. So, it was not a surprise when you continued that same theme right through the diagnosis of cancer and beyond. But I'm aware that some of your closest friends were surprised that you would embrace that approach. They thought you were just trying to be brave. After all, you were diagnosed with CANCER! They seemed to align with their projected fears of possible pain and suffering you might endure, rather than the truth of where you actually were emotionally and philosophically. How could they not know this about you after seeing you live this way for years and years?*

Ah, yes. They love me dearly, and they've seen me this way for years, but they just don't get it. They are beginning to get it, but most just thought that I had a charmed life. They thought I was positive because I had no problems. They'd think, "Well, she's got everything. She's got a wonderful husband, and a wonderful career, and a wonderful..." They didn't realize all of those were also choices. They didn't realize that I would choose to view a diagnosis of cancer the very same way that I had chosen my life prior to that. And for the most part, there's no exception to my perception!

*You took your package of truth into a new arena.*

A new arena. That's right. You know about my mom, right?

*I know many things about her, but tell me more.*

My mother has an amazing spirit. I grew up watching this woman (my mother) who continued to have such a triumphant spirit right through the holocaust and beyond. I mean she danced with people in the camps. And she laughed. She knew you have to laugh. She saved many people's lives because she just wasn't going to take the feelings engendered by that event seriously. Certainly she took the event seriously, because she saved the lives of many people. She helped people escape from camp.

Before going to the camps she took in orphans and fed them. She dared to even go out and take food to other people who were in hiding. She was even kidnapped by the French Resistance because they caught her doing things for Jews hiding in France. Here was this blond, Jewish woman walking around...and she just decided, "I'm just going to walk around and do this!" And she did. I mean, you know—"Nothing will happen to me." So I grew up watching an incredible model of that. It was tough as a teenager, because my mother was very flamboyant about it. *[laughter]* But as a teenager, it's like, "Augh, mom." You know. I was so embarrassed about my mother's boldness.

But, my father based his philosophy of life on the Jewish Talmud. And one of the things he used to repeat, "Who is the happy person? He who chooses 'what is.'" That 'what is' is also a choice. You can think, "Ohmigosh, this befell me." Or you can say, "Yes, it is here, it befell me, and now I'm choosing it."

And so I have to say that a lot of this profound joyfulness and philosophy came directly from these two people. You know, in the Talmud it says there are only two things you get, pain and joy. When it hurts, cry; when it's joyful, laugh. That's basically what I got in my home. So I think that, you know, over the years I've really integrated a very joyful, celebrative, positive, welcoming attitude towards life and all of its events. It has been a part of me to know that it's all blessings.

*It's all "cookies"!*

Yes! Another version of "cookies." And all of the cookies carry a potential blessing. And that's what I've taught.

*And it's your style.*

And it's my style. It's who I am and how I live my life. I think, to be able to apply all of this to cancer, given all that's in the culture about cancer, was a revelation to me. See, it was a revelation, because for six hours on that first day when we got the diagnosis, I was not celebrating. I panicked, and I got really concerned and confused. But it didn't take more than six hours, and I said, "Wait a minute, the news is over, and now it's an event. How am I going to really welcome this event, and what am I going to do?" It was because of the philosophy passed on to me, and subsequently the philosophy I grew to embrace that helped me to remember who I was, even in the face of a diagnosis of cancer. It was also the incredible support from friends like you and Louise. I mean, things like the fact that my dear friend, Louise, fielded all of the phone calls so that I didn't get burdened with any of them. That was fantastic because I was thinking of the stories I could have listened to that would've really—

*Taken you down the wrong road. (Stick end, stick end!)*

Yes, taken me down the wrong road. So it was an amazing realization to me that I could apply this to cancer. And to be able to say, "No, it isn't horrible. It is what it is, and I'm choosing it. It's in my life. I'm choosing it."

*Yeah. Even better, you're choosing your perception of it.*

Yes, I'm choosing my perception of it. And I chose what kind of energy I am going to invest in it, and how I am going to connect with the people who will support my perception and my decision. And that's why I was absolutely dancing when I got your letter.

## Not Why, but "How!"

It came to me that a wonderful title would be "Not WHY, but HOW!" Not why did I get this, and why is this happening to me, and why didn't I know this before, and why, why, why...but "how" am I going to embrace this, and how am I going to welcome it, how am I going to dance with it...you know, all the "hows" that are truly helpful. I'm telling you this, because of the following story. This is truly amazing.

You know, I've been looking for the perfect dress for our son's wedding. And Yumi knows that one of my very favorite things is to go into a store that has fabulous clothes, try everything on and parade around in all the fun, whirling and twirling in delight. And he knows that now it is especially important for me to feel gorgeous, while I am also bald! So after the fourth dose of chemo-therapy, we went on a little get-away to Colorado. We found this beautiful little town called Beaver Creek. It has a fabulous store that could be dubbed "Hedy's Dream Shop." It's absolutely the cat's meow when it comes to clothing. I mean they have every collection of "art-to-wear" type of clothing. The prices are beyond description because that whole area is unbelievably pricey. To my delight, the store had a large array of Blue Fish designs, which is a clothing line that I absolutely adore. They're such unique, wonderful designs. Well, in no time at all, I found this really fabulous dress that was on sale...AND was also a dress that I have no sensible use for! *[laughter]* You know, there are clothes that you absolutely do not need. This is one of them, but it was on sale. It was originally $520.00, which wouldn't be $520.00 anywhere else, but in Beaver Creek it is $520.00. It was reduced half price, and then a little bit more. And I put it on, and absolutely fell in love with myself in it! I just whirled around in the store. And as I'm doing that, this woman approached me, and she said, "I couldn't help but notice that you don't have your hair. Is it chemotherapy?" And I said, "Yes." And she said, "Oh," and she told me her whole story with cancer and her sister's story with cancer.

And as we are talking, this other woman came over and said, "You know, I've just gone through radiation therapy, and I live in Philadelphia, and let me just tell you a little bit about it." And before you knew it, we had this little support group in the middle of the store yakking away and laughing.

*Laughing, that's a key ingredient in any support group!*

Well, the manager of the store overheard us. Of course, we were so loud that you couldn't help but hear us!

*Right. Right, right.*

And each one of us had a new dress on with tags dangling as we visited. Yumi was just laughing at the sight. Then the manager came over, and she said, "Listen, the owner of the store, whom we all love and adore, was just diagnosed with breast cancer yesterday. Would you talk to her on the phone?"

I said, "But of course."

So, I'm talking to her on the phone. And at the very end of our conversation, I said, "Now remember, every cell in your body is already saying, 'I am excited. I am healthy. I am balanced.'"

She said, "And you are healthy yourself? Ooh, it's just so good to talk to you." She said, "Would you talk to my husband? My husband is there in Beaver Creek, but I am at our other home in Evergreen. Would you talk to my husband? He's an engineer, and he has a lot of questions. I can't imagine a better couple than you and your husband to talk to him."

I said, "Of course."

So at 4:30 that afternoon, we met him around the corner in the deli of the Hyatt. He was a lovely, lovely man but distraught— so distraught. He started to tell us about his wife's diagnosis. He said that they have seven children, and that they had recently lost one in a construction accident. A beautiful family; beautiful guy.

And he said, "My wife has been asking why this had to happen, and wondering if it was because of the estrogen she's been on."

And I stopped him right there. I said, "Yumi and I learned very early that putting any energy into 'why' is wasted. Instead, we put our energy into how are we going to do this? How are we going to welcome it today?" And, "How are we going to say 'Yes' to health?"

He said, "Oh, thank you. That is so helpful."

Anyway, he wanted to hear our whole story. When we were finished, he stood up, and he said, "Can I hug you?"

And I said, "Of course!" *[laughter]* And we had this big, big hug. And then he hugged Yumi, as well, and we said goodbye.

During our visit, the store manager dropped by with papers that she gave to him to give his wife, and she said to Yumi, "If you come back for that dress, I'm going to give you a deal you can't refuse!" Well, Yumi and I talked about the dress, and you know, Yumi is very practical. He said, "What are you going to do with that dress? It's probably just going to hang in your closet." And I said, "I don't know, but I can see myself wearing it to synagogue with a hat. I see myself"—you know, I was already dreaming about that dress. Well, I tried to let it go, because I thought, "You know, I really don't want to get something that I wouldn't use," but at the same time I was still dreaming about it. Well, the day before we left we talked about it again, and Yumi said, "Let's go back and get that dress for you." Judie, she gave it to us for $25!

## *Not Why, but "How!"*

Not "why" did I get this? or
"why" is this happening to me? or
"why" didn't I know this before? etc.

But..."How" am I going to embrace this? and
"How" am I going to welcome it?

"How" am I going to dance with it?

(All the "hows" that are really helpful.)

[laughter] A $520 dress for twenty-five dollars! A total gift. And it was out of complete gratefulness for what we had shared. We helped them both to step into that event differently.

*You massaged their perception.*

So that's very exciting. Now, we also told her husband about the sentinel node biopsy. He was very excited about it, but when they talked to the surgeons in Denver, they got a reaction similar to the one doctor that told me: "You're too special for that." They said, "This is too new. Your wife is..." You know, it's going to be standard care in ten years, why not have it now? But that's something that you can't push. It has to be their decision.

*Remember how you felt your way along until you felt confident that you had the perfect plan for you? It doesn't really matter which choice they make. They need to feel good about the entire package, the package they resonate to.*

Exactly. Exactly.

*But, most people are unconsciously responding to energy coming from mass consciousness. Just like when you went to Sarasota for your first (chemo) therapy, there was so much "fear energy" still hovering from all of the people who sat in the same chair before you. Even the term "chemotherapy" has a vibration of fearfulness and vulnerability in it. A commonly held vision about chemotherapy is that it is "attacking" and killing the cancer. Just like the friend who recently said to me, "I know you think you can transmute the side-effects of the chemotherapy, but I don't agree. It is a POISON! And your body is in a major upheaval." As long as that is the perception being held, the likelihood of revolting symptoms is very high.*

*You had anti-nausea medication several times during the first round of "therapy," and it still didn't prevent the violent vomiting. But, as you shifted your perspective, you had no further vomiting following subsequent treatments. You learned to welcome it. You handled the therapy better and better in proportion to your ability to welcome it fully.*

Mm-hmm. That alignment is just so important. Deciding what you will say "Yes" to!

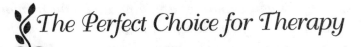

## The Perfect Choice for Therapy

*There must be an ongoing alignment
with whatever therapeutic plan you choose.
From then on, your work is to stay
in alignment as you proceed.
You must feel your way along
using your emotional guidance system.*

## The Gift of Perception

*As I've said before, perception is truly the only thing we have control over.*

Absolutely.

*Your perception is a choice. For example:*

- *Your mother chose how she would perceive the guards in the concentration camps and the director of the refugee camp... deciding to speak to the "human being" in each one instead of speaking to the uniform.*

- *You chose how you would view all therapy relating to your diagnosis.*

- *You chose how you would perceive the diagnosis of cancer... as a temporary "cellular challenge."*

- *A person in pain can choose to embrace thoughts of delight and comfort, and recall enjoyable events. Any pleasurable moment massages the body towards well-being. Pleasurable thoughts provide a cellular tonic.*

- *When a person dies, loved ones can choose to embrace their ongoing invisible presence, or their loss. One is connecting and healing; the second holds them in a state of pain.*

- *When there's been a stormy relationship prior to someone dying, you can choose to draw on who they really were (the wonderful times) or continue the pain of dredging up awful memories. If there literally were no wonderful times, then you can choose to "fill in the blanks," the way it would have been if they had been "connected" to their real selves. You can watch for others who are exemplifying what you would like to have had, and fill in the blanks with that.*

You're absolutely right. Those are powerful choices!

*A few years ago, I was visiting a dear friend who had cancer and was in a lot of pain. She had been addicted to drugs years ago and was concerned that she might become addicted to the pre-scribed pain medication, so she was trying to do without. One thing that she and I had in common was our passion for flowers and gardening. During our visit, we began reminiscing about our favorite northern flowers—flowers that don't grow in Florida! We*

*took turns naming our favorites and groaning together in delight
after each offering.*

*I said, "Lilacs!" and we'd go, "OOOOOOOOH!"*
*And she said, "Lily of the Valley!" "OOOOOOOOH!"*
*"Snowball Bushes!" "OOOOOOOH!"*
*"Daffodils!" "OOOOOOOOH!"*

*And we just kept taking turns. We must have named at least
forty favorites. When we were through, her pain had all but
disappeared. That's daffodil power for you! Actually, it's the
power of purposeful perception. What a tonic.*

That's fabulous!

*About a year later, my friend passed away peacefully, just hours
after I had whispered a wonderful list to her of flowers she'd
surely find in Heaven. I whispered visions of her transition being
the sensation of stepping out of a stuffy room and into wonderfully fresh air. That it would be like stepping out of tight shoes,
and into fluffy bedroom slippers. Just 10 minutes before her
passing, she assured the nurse that she was quite comfortable.
She was aligned with a perception of the very best life here, and
her fabulous life on the other side that would soon follow. It was
an effortless, alert and joy-filled transition. The magical ingredient was perception.*

You know, we need to remember we have options. Reality changes
as we change our perception of that reality.

*Exactly. As a matter of fact, her 24-year-old daughter had many
unpleasant memories of times with her mother and was "stuck"
in "what was." She was growing up during the time her mother
had been on drugs and alcohol. She had never worked through
the bitterness that stemmed from those years. Relationships are
eternal. Her mother was now physically gone, and she was still
choosing to reference the worst part of their time together. Once
again, the shift to peace is as close as your shift in perception.*

*There's a "loving self" and an "ornery self" inside each of us to some degree, as our valve to well-being and Authenticity opens and closes. We have the option, even after someone in our life dies, to choose which version we will focus on within the invisible relationship that continues right on. We have the option of saying, "I forgive you for not being the person I wanted you to be." You might as well find a version of them that pleases you, and enjoy yourself. They are! You are the only one that your unloving thoughts are taking a toll on. The person you adore is just a perception away.*

### Thoughts to Ponder...

*Relationships are eternal.*
*Perception is a choice.*

*So whether it is something on the news, a person who has hurt you, people in authority who can potentially make your life miserable, an offsetting diagnosis, or the loss of a loved one (or unloved one), the salve for the soul is your choice of perception! The teacher and healer known as Jesus Christ said, "Turn the other cheek!" In other words, look in a different direction to find another way of perceiving the situation. Ask the empowering question, "What's another way I can see this?"*

### Salve for Every Soul

*Listen to (or find) the music*
*of the past in order to sing in the present*
*and dance into the future.*
*~Unknown*

# *Pondering My Next Role with the Kosher Choreographer!*
### *(Ready...and "Action!")*

You know, on Valentine's Day, just prior to my mammogram and the diagnosis that followed, Yumi and I were sitting having a drink after work. Suddenly this sentence came through me...it was that, "If I died right now, the world is different because I've walked through it." I just burst out crying, and I told Yumi what I had heard inside my head. I just cried and cried, but it was like, "What's going on with Hedy?" I said to Yumi, "I don't know what's going on with me, but I really feel if I should die right now, I've made a real difference, and that's just wonderful to know."... And, you know, like that. And then I said, "I'm curious as to how I'm going to be used, now that I know that. And what my next contribution will be."

*Mm-hmm.*

Following that, we went to visit my friend Linda, you know, my friend who had the diagnosis of terminal cancer, and who is now fabulously well. (So well that now she wants to come and visit me!) Anyway, we went to visit her, and it was the first time Yumi had seen her since her recovery. He was just so amazed. She talked to Yumi about just "grabbing life" and "being happy for every moment." She said some very sweet things. But the irony was, that I chose to go see her that evening...a person, who miraculously just stepped out of what people would describe as having been at "death's door." You'll remember she was in a coma, 90 pounds, and we fully expected her to die any moment. And then she like "stepped out of it," and there she was. After asking myself the question, "How am I going to be used now? Let's see what shows up now in my life," she was the person I went to see that night. And the next thing that shows up in my life is a personal diagnosis of breast cancer. Is that phenomenal? And the whole journey that followed!

*"Journey" is certainly the operative word. You saw it as a journey and one to be lived fully as you moved along your path. You were never just enduring, "waiting," or in a "holding pattern" until you could get on with your life.*

Mm-hmm, mm-hmm, mm-hmm. An incredible journey! I certainly got my answer to, "How am I going to be used next?!"

# Chapter 16

# Soul Illumination

## RRRRRadiation Therapy

Soon after I began radiation therapy, I told Yumi, "I'm rrrrrra-diating!" We got such a big laugh out of the vision of me, glowing more and more with each treatment. Naturally, this was one more time that I asked the staff if I could have Yumi at my side, and he was once again allowed to come in. We promptly made friends with two women on each side of me and saw them regularly on each visit. We formed a little community and when each of them was finished with their course of radiation, we all said warm good-byes and "we'll miss you." It was very nice.

On my first visit, the nurses wanted a picture of me for identification purposes, as part of my chart. And so, when they requested the picture, I said, "Oh, a picture? If there is going to be a picture, I want it with my husband!" *[laughter]* So Yumi got in on the picture. And now there's this picture of the two of us on my chart. Well, the staff really got a kick out of this. Every time they'd open my chart, they'd laugh because it's unusual to see a "couple" smiling back at them. *[laughter]* And they said this has been so wonderful for them. You know, whenever they need to laugh, they open up our chart and there is that picture of the two of us. So funny, so funny. *[reminiscing]:* The bold, the bald and...the beautiful Yumi! Very, very funny.

Oh, I almost forgot that they took a second picture. Each time we pulled the curtain so that I could get undressed, Yumi was with me behind the curtain. They took a candid picture of our feet! These "four feet" running around under the curtain. They even got a kick out of that sight.

*Kodak moments! [laughing]*

Yes, it was wonderful.

## Angela and the Magical Bear

I must tell you about a profound part of my experience there. When I first began radiation, I noticed something very interesting. Initially, it ran like clockwork. I arrived at 3:45 p.m., they'd give me a gown, I'd have my treatment, and that was that. Then, slowly but surely, they were later and later.

On the next appointment I showed up at 3:45 p.m. but this time there were new people on either side of me, and they were on stretchers. One was a teenage girl who apparently had throat cancer. But, at that point, I wasn't willing to interact with either of them...instead I was focused on the fact that now it was 3:55 p.m. and that no one had come!

*You began giving your full attention to the delay. Valve closed, valve closed!*

Exactly. Now it is 4:05...and I'm thinking "this person is on the stretcher and it will take a long time," and I'm silently "huffin' and puffin' inside" about the delay. Well, the father of the little girl suddenly appeared and eagerly came over saying, "Hi, I'm Rob, and this is my daughter Angela! It's so nice to see you..." and all of that. And he continued, "You have become a topic of conversation in our family!" I said, "Really?" And he said, "Yes, you have, and I just wanted to thank you for that. You were here when we were visiting for the very first time. You came in with your bald head. I said, 'Angela, look at that lady...she's just proudly walking around with her bald head...(you know) It's just like she's saying, look at me folks!' I said, 'See, Angela, you could do that too!' We were so inspired by you. We laughed and laughed about the wonderful bald-headed lady!"

I thought, "Wow." You know, it never occurred to me that my baldness was inspiring anyone, and that I could be the topic of a conversation about it.

*Are you kidding?!*

No! I had never thought of that. Well, needless to say, I was no longer tapping my foot and noticing the time.

*They enticed you back into connection, just like you and Yumi do with so many.*

Exactly...I was reconnected. And I thought, "When Angela comes out, I want to make a connection with her."

So when she came out, I went over to her (knowing she is unable to speak) and said, *[melodically]*: "Angela, we share the same hard table! And today, you warmed it up for me...tomorrow, I might warm it up for you!" and she smiled, you know. So she left. And the next day indeed, I warmed it up for her. She was waiting when I came out. I said, "Angela, I warmed it up for you!"

So that night, while lying in bed awake, I suddenly noticed the magical little bear named "Wanda" that you had given to me to help keep my "valve" wide open. I thought, I'm going to give this bear to Angela. And I'm going to tell her that this is a magical bear, which it is, that I don't need it anymore, and that I'm passing it on to her. And when she doesn't need it anymore, she can pass it on to the next person! And I thought that I would include a note about what a beautiful, courageous person she is. I used some pretty stationery...some long sheets that say, "At night, I give all my worries to God because He's going to be up all night anyway!" I wrote, "Dear Angela, this is a magical bear," etc., and I wrote the whole thing 'cause I didn't know if I would get to see her personally that day.

So, the next day, I took "Wanda" the bear, with me. But, when we arrived, Angela wasn't there. I received my treatment and Angela still wasn't there. And I asked the staff where she was and they said her father called and said that she would be late today. Yumi said (to me), "Well, we can give her the bear tomorrow." And I said, "No...we have to give her the bear today...I don't know why but we have to wait for her." So we waited—and this "patient me" was so strikingly different from the "huffin' and puffin' me" that previously noted, "It's five to four and no one has come!" Now I was casually saying, "Hey, let's just wait for Angela!" You know, it's so funny, once you make "the connection"...you shift to "eternal time!"

*So well put...You slide right into "eternal time!" [uproarious laughter] It's a mere "perception" away.*

### Eternal Time!

*So we waited—and this "patient me"*
*was so strikingly different from the*
*"huffin' and puffin' me" that previously noted,*
*"It's five to four and no one has come!"*
*You know, it's so funny, once you make*
*"the connection"...*
*you shift to "eternal time!"*
*It's a mere "perception" away!*

Exactly. So Angela finally arrived. You know, she was on oxygen, on a stretcher, and had nurses all around her. I went over and said, "Angela, I brought you something. I have a little bear here that's a magical bear! It was given to me to help me when I needed it. I don't need it anymore, so I want you to have it. And, when you don't need this bear anymore, you just give it to the next person." She started to cry, and she whispered, "Thank you." And I said, "You're very welcome." I said, "Give me five." And she did. I said, "Wow, you have a lot of energy in there!"

*Oh, perfect.*

Well, I went back yesterday, and the staff said, "What did you do to Angela with that bear? She got off the stretcher!" She <u>walked</u> into the room! *[exuberantly]:* I said smiling, "I don't know." It's just a magical bear.

*Whooooah! Goose bumps! On a "goose bump index" (GBI), it got the maximum of 10! It's a 10! That means no goose left un-bumped! [laughing] What a moment!*

*[laughter]* A GBI of 10! That's perfect!
  Now, the other piece in this story that is quite interesting is that, prior to that day, Angela always had a little stuffed dog with her. And that day they accidentally forgot the dog.

*Oh, wow. That's just fabulous. We are easily entertained, aren't we? [laughing]*

*[reflectively]:* She forgot the dog. I mean, her father forgot the dog, and—

*Yeah. Major synchronicity.*

Somehow I knew I had to give it to her that day. Isn't that an amazing story about that bear? That's the little "energized" bear you brought to me that night that I was in bed with a fever. That little guy was just packed with energy...just packed with energy. Packed. She held that bear and it got her off her stretcher!

*More accurately, you and "Wanda" connected Angela with her Core Energy, empowering her. That's when miracles happen. The two of you helped her open her valve! What a timely, loving gesture.*

Oh, yes. Oh, yes. As she read the note, I could see how much she embraced what I had written. There's not much verbal communication with her. People don't approach her. She's bloated, she doesn't look like Angela. But underneath there, of course, is Angela going, "Hello out there, I'm in here. Please acknowledge me."

I chuckled as I arrived for my next treatment, and had let go of all resistance about them not keeping a timely schedule. Absolutely no other patients were there. The coast was totally clear, as if deliberately choreographed for my ease. I mean, it was so amazing to see. And to add to that, on this day, the nurses were sharing fresh-baked apple and cherry pie that someone had brought as a gift. And of course, my treatment went like clockwork. We arrived—we were called in—they treated me—we came out—we received delicious cherry pie and apple pie (from the Kosher Choreographer!)—and we were on our way. *[laughter]* We were both radiating! The Kosher Choreographer arranged a celebration, complete with pie. It was so amazing. It's like, you re-establish your balance, and God's angels clear a path so wide, that there's absolutely no one there to delay your tour through the department. I can hear angels saying, "You want a path...we'll show you a path! And we'll even throw in pie!" That's exactly how I saw it. It's was just phenomenal. The Kosher Choreographer at work again.

*Heavenly servings of pie! [laughing]*

It was delicious.

One by one, we met a number of fascinating women having radiation treatments. They were in various stages of whatever diagnosis they had. I noticed one woman that just wouldn't make any eye contact with me, no matter what. So I finally thought, this requires more of a connection than "Well, hello, I'm Hedy." So, one day she was sitting there, and I just sat down next to her, and I said, "You know, you and I have really been doing this thing together, for quite some time now, and I just wanted to say hi." And to my delight, her whole face broke into a smile. She said, "Oh, hi." And I said, "How's it going?" And she said, "Well, this is going well," she said, "but my life is not." And I said, "Oh." And she said, "Well, when I got this diagnosis of cancer I also lost my job, and, you know, I'm not young... and that presents problems in getting another job. And... now I also have a problem about my insurance, since it was through my work." And she began to really spill her heart about how hopeless she felt. And, I just really listened to her, and said, "Well, you know, that's really a lot to carry because, I mean, just the diagnosis of cancer and all that it immediately involves, is a trip by itself!" And I said, "To add to that, the idea of not having a job right now, that's a lot. I am just in awe that you are here every day, just doing your thing. I'm in awe!" We chatted just a little more and then we said our good-bye.

So, every time we went to my appointment, we greeted her warmly and chatted a bit. Then she came to the end of her treatment, and I said, "You know, I come from a tradition where people bless people," and I said, "I'm just going to bless you! I bless you with a very fulfilling, wonderful job that just is the best thing you could dream of. And I bless you with wonderful health, vitality and joy. That is my blessing." And she said, "Oh gosh, from your mouth to God's ears." I mean, it was just a lovely connection. And that was it.

*There you go again, performing another "valve job!" First Angela, and now this woman. You helped to empower both of them. That's what healing is all about... opening back up to what never went away! Instead of joining their pain, you acted as a touchstone for greater things. You helped them click right back into place!*

That's it. CLICK! CLICK! CLICK! CLICK!

## *Another "Valve Job!"*

*There you go again, performing another
"valve job!" First Angela, and now this woman.
You helped to empower both of them.
That's what healing is all about...
opening back up to what never went away!*

*<u>Instead of joining their pain,</u>
you acted as
a touchstone for greater things.
You helped them click right back into place!*

# *The Inconsolable Place!*

Well, I returned to a very old place this past week. Only this time, I was finally able to name it, and consequently it became a new place with a new perspective. It felt familiar and yet new—old and young at the same time. I called it the "unsupportable place" because it really is like when you were a baby... you're just so uncomfortable and...

*Inconsolable!*

That's it. Inconsolable! And, you know, you are beyond the threshold of your own endurance, and that's exactly where I was. It was partially due to sleep deprivation...I was very tired. I've slept a little better since then.

*It was probably sleeplessness caused by that "new hair" growing in the night. The noise was keeping you awake!*

*[laughter]* That's it...my new hair—growing! It was also the burning sensation from the radiation...it was everything I could list that wasn't the way I wanted it. (Valve closed.) I took it all

with me into "that place." The beauty is, that I know I don't have to explain about it... I just have to cry. You know... it's such a nice thing to know that I just have to cry, and cry, and cry, and be like that little baby that just lets it all out. So I did.

*Were you by yourself?*

Yes, I was by myself because Yumi went to his men's group. The funny thing was that Yumi had asked, "Do you want me to stay with you?" I said, "No." *[pouting]* He said, "Are you sure?" "Yep." *[more pouting]*

*[laughing] We need video tape of you telling this!*

So he left. Then I began blubbering about that to myself! I added it to my list. "He left! He didn't stay with me!" But then he soon returned. I thought for a moment that he was coming back to stay with me... but he had merely forgotten his car keys. He picked up his keys, and then left again! *[laughter]* You know! But, his staying with me was not the answer. I truly needed to just embrace this place I was in, and release it through tears. If he would have stayed, he would have felt so helpless... even he wouldn't have been able to console me. Whatever he offered would have been the wrong thing. If he came close: "You're crowding me." If he gave me some space: "You're abandoning me." If he just stood there: "Do something!" etc. You know, I was "inconsolable!" So I let the tears just flow and flow.

It was so amazing to feel the change in me as I cried it out, and just let it out. Afterwards, I felt so wonderful. And now that I have been able to give it a name, I've made friends with it. I welcome it and let it flow right on through me, and right on out through my tears.

*The inconsolable place—you feel it, name it, embrace it, and surrender to it... then release it with your tears. That's great.*

You know, to know to just say, "Okay...it's the inconsolable, unsupportable place. I know just what to do for this, and no one can do it for me. I must do it myself." Later, when Yumi and I talked about it, he admitted that he was grateful to be off to his men's group, because he really didn't know what to do for the "inconsolable" me.

*But, you know, you truly set the intention for what it was you were doing. You were crying with your focus on the release, or as author Iyanla Vanzant puts it, you were "crying with an agenda."[1] That's a lot different from crying unending tears as you continue to focus on the problem or problems, or crying to a mantra of "ain't it awful" as you recycle pain and frustrations. In your case, you were making your way to the light. You gradually freed yourself from the toilet paper that was stuck to your foot. Nice release!*

Yes! Thank you! It delivered a fresh new "me" that felt wonderful!

## *The Credit Department*

You know, ever since I began radiation, I've been using this cream called Biafine Cream. Even the nurses can't get over how well my skin is doing. They said that the cream seems to have made an extraordinary difference. At least something has. Most people are cracked and inflamed after radiation. I have only the slightest redness.

*Your skin does look great.*

The nurses said that I have provided some valuable research data for them by using it. Because, from what they're seeing, my skin is really quite remarkable.

*A real research project would be to divide your breast down the middle and just use it on half of the breast. [laughing]*

## *Crying with an Agenda!*

*You truly set the intention for what it
was you were doing. You were crying
with your focus on the <u>release</u>.
That's a lot different from crying
unending tears as you continue to focus
on the problem or problems.
In your case, you were making your way to the light!
You gradually freed yourself from the toilet paper
that was stuck to your foot.*

*Nice release!*

Half of the breast. You know, at this point, if they want to do something with it, they'll have to—

*Find someone else! [giggling]*

I am very glad I used it as religiously as I did, and now I'm going to continue to really pamper this wonderful little breast. It has gone through quite a bit.

*While I understand that the cream may have worked wonders, I still want you to consider the larger picture. You have continually lived in a way that has promoted this unbelievable flow of Life Force. Take for example, all the celebrating you took part in. Every cell was responding to that joy. It's so powerful, but also invisible. Because we can "see and feel" cream, it's so much easier to have a belief in the cream.*

In the cream, yes.

*And so, I'll let you give credit to the cream, and I'm going to give major credit to all the ways you found to stay fully open to the flow of Life Force. Your belief in the cream played a supporting role in that flow. The cream paired with celebration is just so powerful! Whatever works, works! Opening your valve to the flow of Life Force is the most powerful medicine in the Kosher Choreographer's pharmacy! If you were to use the cream while continually banging your way through life with a lot of resistance, I'm willing to bet the results wouldn't have been as dramatic. You might want to give credit where credit is due! You played the greatest leading role in the process. The cream played a supportive role as a wonderful valve-opener.*

Exactly. I'll take God's pharmacy any day!

You know, a few days ago, I spotted Angela in the ambulance after I hadn't seen her for some time. So I crawled in there. I was telling the story to the staff and they said to me today, "You know, I don't know anyone else who would have crawled into that ambulance." They said, "She looks forward to seeing you. There is something about the way you greet her. We've noticed that she waits to see if you're going to be there on that day," and so on, and so on. So, you know, it's becoming clearer that my own happiness really permeates all my cells, and other people's cells.

*It's the gift that keeps on giving!*

Precisely.

Today the staff said they had never seen patients go around the unit saying "hello" to everybody. You know, it's just been such a nice arena to simply be in awe of life. You can focus on disease, or you can be in awe of life and the amazing people who are showing up. It's as simple as that. "Awe" is wonderfully portable. We can even take it into the radiation oncology department. You can be in "awe" of life, everywhere!

Well, I am ready now to hop on your table to embrace your artistry...so get those nuclear hands warmed up for another fabulous therapeutic treatment! Uhmmmmm.

## *It's Your Call!*

*You can focus on disease, or you can be
in awe of life. It's just as simple as that!
"Awe" is wonderfully portable. We can even take
it into the radiation oncology department!
You can be in "awe" of life, everywhere!*

# *It's Chest Admiration!*

Well, I must tell you that I went for my checkup, and they could not believe the way my breast looks. It looks just like the other one; the color and the quality of the skin is just wonderful. The scar is nearly invisible. They couldn't believe it...this is one month after the last radiation treatment. The nurse said, never in her whole career had she ever seen anyone do this well. And I said, "It's love, it's love." *[teasingly]:* "It's love, and it's the cream I use." She said she wanted to know about the cream.

*I was hoping she'd want to know about the love! [teasing]*

Yes...look how quickly love is passed over for something (like a cream) that you can sink your fingers into! But the examination was really quite extraordinary and, of course, my mammogram was perfect.

# *Reflections*

*What new vision has this whole journey given you?*

You know, two major elements framed not only this journey, but my whole life. One is the understanding that "news" is only news for a very short time, and then it's not news anymore. So when it's news, it's either good or bad. But when it's done being news, it's an event. And the event is to be welcomed completely, with everything we have to offer to it, for the growth of our soul. It was very empowering for Yumi and me to know that. So that was one enormous "message."

*Perceiving it all as an event, brings it down to size and makes it easier for you to focus your energy.*

Right. Right. The news then becomes an event, and now we bring to it everything we are, up to today. The event is in our life to grow our soul. There is no other reason that this event is in our life. So now, how are we going to welcome it so that we have maximum benefit for our soul?

And then the second big thing that is so clear is that "God has given us time and space, and then it's our job to fill it with joy and meaning." Clearly! I mean that's up to us. God does not give us joy and meaning; WE create joy and meaning. Time and space is a huge gift already. In this journey, we were even more aware that we had a lot of time, because we stopped all the other things we were doing. You know, I'm the first to admit that I didn't feel physically good, all the time. But even when I was feeling physically bad, I was feeling spiritually outstanding. I was still embracing the bigger picture!

*What a profound statement!*

 ## The Power of Connection

*You know, I'm the first to admit
that I didn't feel physically good, all the time.*
**But even when I was feeling
physically bad,
I was feeling spiritually outstanding.**
*I was still embracing the bigger picture!*

So that's a pretty incredible thing to be able to witness! It's been wonderful to see the real distinction between, "Yes, my body is really 'busy' and uncomfortable right now, but my spirit is soaring." It's similar to that story of when I was vomiting in the car after my first therapy...the way you guided us to our destination with your beautiful words of imagery and I was able to mentally slide into my bed before we had arrived. Even through the misery I was able to enjoy better times to come, in advance. I was physically more uncomfortable than I've ever been, and spiritually I was acknowledging, "Oh, my God, this is amazing! Look what's happening. There is this voice, your heavenly voice, coming into the car." It was absolutely magical.

*Oh, yes.*

## The Message of the Journey

*The message in all of this, is that it is up to us to fill time and space with joy and meaning. A diagnosis of cancer becomes an event, for the growth of our souls. We need to ask ourselves what we are going to do with it, and how are we going to celebrate and welcome this event.*

As I stated before, I don't plan on "doing cancer" again, so I might as well do it WELL! Like the couple I spoke to in Colorado who were just one day into the diagnosis when they met us. He said their whole energy went into "why," thinking that by understanding the "why" they can prevent it from happening again. They thought surely she must have been doing something wrong, or she wouldn't have gotten it. You know, I spoke to them again recently, and they said that not asking "why" but instead asking "how" was absolutely life changing. It absolutely empowered them. They are both doing very well.

*That's just fabulous!*

I've come to know that "all is as it should be" and to reign in my energy on the subject. It was so clear to me that whenever our energy even slightly focused on "why," we would say, *[in a sing-song, matter-of-fact tone]:* "Un-necessary!" We are not privy to the mystery of life. We just are not. It is not our job to understand it; it is our job to live it. And as we live it, we come to know pieces of it, but the whole mystery is not for us to know. It is for us to be in awe of! And that is another thing that was very clear. I'll never fully understand this thing. Might as well relax about it. This is "what is" in my life. This too, is packed with opportunities. As you said, "It's a gift wrapped in breast tissue!" That's it.

*Yeah, relax and just concentrate on keeping your valve open. Any time you are focused on the "why," you're also at the stick end of the wand and have diminished well-being. You've diminished the very ingredient your cells are calling for. Thinking that you must have done something wrong—also pairs you with the stick end of the wand.*

*[mimicking and pointing a finger]:* You did something **wrong!**

*You, on the other hand, in your focus on doing this thing "well," put your whole attention on living each moment as fully connected to Source energy as you could possibly be. You deliberately chose things that promoted and celebrated good health. It would be more accurate to say that you focused on "Health" with a capital "H," which equates to Spirit or soul. All of that simultaneously kept you at the star end of the wand, where Life Force or God Force flows abundantly. Right where you need to be, to reclaim your perfect health.*

Exactly. Right where you need to be. *[quietly and with certainty]:* Yes, yes, yes. I also had ongoing spiritual confidence that everything I needed for this journey would be provided for me...and that has truly been the case. But, I couldn't have recognized what had been provided, without being at the star end of the wand. The welcoming, surrendering, celebrating, releasing, appreciating, trusting, laughing…all played major roles in allowing me to see where to step next on this journey.

I love to say two things to people. One is a take-off on the cliché: "God doesn't close a door without opening another one." I've added: "Yes, and it's fucking dark in the corridor in the meantime!" *[howling with laughter]* And just knowing that it's "fucking dark in the corridor meanwhile" is really quite nice, because you know the door is going to open. So let's just welcome the darkness. In the meantime, you know, you're just in the corridor. I think that that's been a really nice one for me now, knowing that because I trust guidance, and "guidance comes…when guidance comes!" *[unable to resist saying it one more time, repeated in an arpeggio style]:* "The door is going to open, but it's **fucking dark, and it's fine!"**

The second thing is one that I have probably told you about. It's an "afge" (pronounced "aff-gee"). A-f-g-e stands for: "Another fucking growth experience!"

*[laughing] Hilarious! Just hilarious!*

### *Another "Hedy-ism"*

*You know the saying,*
*"God doesn't close a door without*
*opening another one." I've added:*
*"Yes, and it's fucking dark*
*in the corridor in the meantime!"*

And this is just so precious because the journey has these moments that truly are "afge's," like when I got that fax about the node that they thought was now malignant. It was in medical terminology, and it looked so awful. That was an "afge" because, one moment we were flying along confidently, and in the next we felt extremely vulnerable.

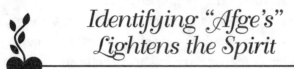

### Identifying "Afge's" Lightens the Spirit

*On a challenging day, remember to say,*
*"Oh, this is another Af-ge!" (pronounced "aff-gee")*
*"Afge" stands for:*

*"Another fucking growth experience!"*

Three additional things that I love to say in my talks are:

• Pain is inevitable, suffering is optional,
   (and really to know the distinction between the two).

• Change is inevitable, growth is optional.

I think those are so profound.

*[laughter] Absolutely! Growth is optional!*

And the third one that I love to say is, "I don't believe in miracles, I rely on them." And I really did. I just relied on the inner knowing that each piece of this journey was going to be completely perfect, that we would meet the perfect people, and find the perfect

### Options!

*Pain is inevitable…suffering is optional!*
*Change is inevitable…growth is optional!*

*More Hedy-ism's!*

*I don't believe in miracles...*
*I rely on them!*

doctor and be in the perfect place and, you know, all of that. Even the "fucking dark corridor" times had their own purpose. The door always opened.

You know, part of my sense of flow in this journey has been my willingness to co-operate with my body's new incarnation, or transformation. When I needed to rest, I rested. When I needed to sleep, I slept. When I needed to eat, I ate. And when I needed to cry, I cried. I love to cry. I love that wonderful feeling afterwards. I cry with my sights set on that. But I have noticed how offsetting my tears always are for those around me. People immediately think they must "do something" about my crying, and the list of things they suggest is rather entertaining. Rather than just getting comfortable with my tears, they suggest that I take a bath, see a movie, eat warm food, read a book, put on music, breathe deeply, go for a walk, etc. I just need to cry! I must do that to take good care of myself, and get to that wonderful feeling that awaits me at the end of the tears.

*Well, I think the important part of this is that you are one who knows how to cry with purpose. Some flail about while fully focused on their misery, and actually need some outer stimulus to get them to the star end of the wand. You are automatically headed there. You could probably be labeled, "A Professional Cryer!" One who knows where the tears are taking her!*

I see what you mean. I do "do it well!" *[laughing]*

I'll tell you something else. I was given a number of audio tapes that were thought to be helpful and positive, but these tapes were truly not helpful. I listened to many of the so-called healing tapes, and their focus was not on embracing the joy of life.

*Unh-uh. Absolutely. Joy is the critical ingredient in being fully alive. It doesn't necessarily mean you're grinning and laughing. (Although laughter and smiles are fabulous.) The Joy you and I are talking about is the state of spiritual connection and spiritual aliveness. It covers a broad range from uproarious, side-splitting laughter to the quiet knowing that all is well—even when your body is very busy or uncomfortable. It's the Joy-filled spirit that seemed to be missing in the tapes that I've listened to. They are mostly about fighting against cancer, or fighting against the problem, instead of embracing a much larger truth...Joy.*

That's it. Fighting against the problem. And the tone in some of them seemed to be soooo solemn, rather than filled with the joy of being alive. You know, you're alive—'til you're dead! I wanted something that celebrated that. One tape that was sent from a wonderful Rabbi had such a solemn tone that it felt like grieving.

*Grieving for...*

For a dead person!

*A dead person! Whoa! [laughter]*

Even the ones by leading authorities still talked of killing the cancer. They still were not embracing the joy of life and the magnificence of the human body. Your tape was the only one I could resonate to...truly a celebration throughout, and so supportive during the therapy. Hopefully, they will continue to gravitate towards tapes like yours, and away from pushing against cancer.

*I think the whole scenario about "killing cancer" came about because people perceive it as being much bigger than they are. It feels like an assault in the night by "something" gigantic. And like a situation in which you ought to grab a weapon to defend yourself. But once you understand illness from the perspective that you've merely pinched off the flow of your well-being, the focus is naturally on what would open this flow back up. It's as simple as "valve closed...valve open," rather than "blow 'em to bits" and "hope we got 'em all"! Some are ready for this perspective and some are not.*

It's truly the only version that I resonate to. I feel the profound truth in the mere thought of "opening myself up to the flow of well-being."

On another note, I had a dream recently in which one of the messages seemed to be about getting a second chance. And this "second chance" is very profound for me...this time of newness and a "new me." This "new me" is really doing things without fear. I've been fearless! I've done three things this week that were big: I taught a completely new training seminar for therapists. During the seminar, a dynamic happened between two people that was very, very difficult, and I just sailed through it. I had no fear!

On Friday, I gave a talk downtown for a group of seventy counselors. Judie, I just stepped into that thing. I looked around and was so taken by the beauty looking back at me. I said, "All of you look so beautiful. I don't think I've ever seen a room full of such handsome people." One girl said, "You must say this to every audience." I said, *[softly and with a grand smile]:* "I don't, but that's not a bad idea!" *[laughter]* Anyway, this thing just flowed. Judie, I had no fear.

Then I performed a wedding ceremony yesterday for a friend. It was a very mixed group. Some of them bikers, professors at the university who are bikers. It appeared to be a unique group that would tend to be a bit cynical about sentimental things. *[lowering her voice to a whisper]:* Well, I stepped into that thing, and it was <u>gorgeous</u>! Many people came to me afterwards saying that this was the most beautiful wedding ceremony they'd ever attended. I had no fear!

Whenever somebody asks me how I'm doing, I say things like, "phenomenal," "clean bill of health," "no cancer anywhere," "I'm done with the thing." After hearing this, Yumi said later, "You can't really say that, because statistically no one ever really knows." I said, "Well, Yumi Schleifer, a 'statistic' is truth with a small 't'—and I'm talking about truth with a big 'T.'" He looked at me, he says, "I know what you mean." *[emphatically and upbeat]:* But it's true. I said, "Because in the future, if I have to face cancer…then I face cancer! I mean, does cancer frighten me? Today, I'm 100% cancer free and well. A hundred percent well. I'm beyond well." I said to Yumi, "And I want you to step into this same program, because I don't want you to have 'that look' on your face that some people have when I say that I'm well, and they say, *[in a tiny, questioning voice]:* 'Really?' Because you have to step into the big Truth. We're not doing small truth here between us!" Yumi said, "You're right. I'll join you in the Big Truth."

So I think that my "new fearless self" paired with the flow of life is just powerful. I mean, I'll face a lot of things in my life and one might be cancer. I don't know. It doesn't matter.
It would just be, as you say, more "cookies!"

*Oh, you're such a quick study.*

Augh, just the next cookie! *[laughter]* Just the next cookie. So, for me, the element of the second time around without fear is priceless.

*Author Wayne Dyer once told a story about life on a planet called "Uranus" where there are different options in life. On that planet, you can opt to go into "rewind" any time you don't like how it played out the first time around. You just instantly rewind any moment or event in life and do it again in a way that suits you better. In a way, that's the option that you've been given; you can return to familiar roles again without the fear.*

Exactly. I've been told that women may grieve for two years after breast surgery. But, I decided that I'm not going to grieve. Instead, I'll celebrate for two years! And after those two years, I'll find another list of things to celebrate. The main thing is that I am finding it more delicious than ever to focus right here in the present and rejoice about life. My standard answer for anything that I don't feel called to do, is "Not now...not for two years." The fun thing is that the two-year mark always (secretly) begins today, so it's a perpetual two years of celebration that will never end. It's an expanded "new me!"

One important part of this "new me" is that I'm also paying attention to appropriate places to use the word "No!" I didn't use that word much in my vocabulary prior to this experience. I am paying attention to where I choose to say "no," and it's doing something wonderful for Yumi and me. Yumi tends to be "future oriented." He's always thinking about, "let's do this and let's do that," and "let's build this in and let's build that in." Lately, I find myself saying, "I want you to hear something for me. *[softly]:* No, not now, not yet." So, I am purposefully saying "No" and then inviting him to join me in the "present."

The other day, I taught this beautiful training seminar. Once I had finished, Yumi was so excited about the training I did, that he suddenly began rattling off a list of future projects I could do. I said, "These are wonderful ideas, but right now, no. This whole evening is for rejoicing about what I just did. Join me in celebrating this day." And he said, "Oh, you're right." And he just pulled his focus back from the future, and he joined me in celebration of the present. And it was beautiful for both of us. When Yumi shoots off into the future, he feels all alone because I don't join him. But actually, I am excited about it with him, but right now, I want him to join me in the present.

So this is a big thing. I say "no" differently now. Before, I would say "no" sometimes as a reaction. *[emphatically]:* "NO!" But not as something that was paired with a "yes." No, I don't want to make plans now...because I want to say "yes" to the celebration of this moment.

*It's the best kind of "no," a "no with a yes!" "I don't care for the peanut butter cookies, but I'll sure have several chocolate chip!"*

Yes. Yes!

*I'm hearing you say, "I choose this instead, thank you." You're not wasting your energy by staying stuck in "no." You're not pushing or resisting, you're just making a choice. You've shifted your focus to what you are wanting to choose. You have energetically paired it with what intuitively feels better.*

This is what I'm choosing. However, I'm choosing to wait on that. I'm choosing to embrace this moment.

*Your "no" is paired with vision. It's a visionary "no"!*

That's it! You know, people invite me to do things all the time, and I am finding myself saying, "No, thank you. I've found that it pays for me to be sensitive to how much I put on my professional plate, and consequently, I must say no. But, thank you for thinking of me."

*What a beautiful "no!" as you said "yes" to a schedule that feels better. A "no with a yes," it's just the best. It's a decision to move forward in a way that suits you, which means it simultaneously increases your feeling of aliveness. It's that rush of energy that always follows a good feeling.*

Yes. It feels wonderful.

The other thing I want to tell you about is really quite extraordinary. In our last workshop, in Fort Lauderdale, we had a phenomenal couple sitting there. I could tell right away that they had done a lot of work, both on their own selves, on their relationship, and on who they are. They were really a powerful, powerful couple. It turned out that the woman is the head of a breast cancer clinic at a medical school. What a synchronistic moment. *[laughter]* And he is the head of the psychoneuroim-munology department of the medical school. So, the first thing I did during the workshop is to tell them that I've just had chemotherapy and so on, and that Yumi and I had learned to welcome this whole journey and make the treatment a friend. Well, they were both so impressed about our approach. She said that this is precisely what they're trying to teach people in their clinic—how to make the treatment a friend. She's found that there are a lot of people who find that really tough, and resist the entire idea of the unlikely friendship. She was saying that they have discovered that the immune system is so precisely modulated that when people pass by the place where they got chemotherapy, their immune system goes down in response to the visual stimulus. Not only that, she said that people will start to feel nauseous, and some people will even vomit, just passing by the building! She said that she ran into a previous chemotherapy patient one day in the supermarket near the cucum-bers, and as soon as the woman saw her, she vomited all over the cucumbers!

*Wow.*

So on the way back, I said to Yumi, "I want to mentally visit all those places and see what happens," you know, see if I'm going to feel nauseous—see if it makes me vomit. You know, all of that. So I went back, in my mind. The first place I visited, was the place where I got the chemotherapy. One day you must see it! It has lots of large windows overlooking an area just like your gorgeous backyard. It's lush and green and has flowers. The sun is shining. The people were, with maybe one or two exceptions, charming, welcoming, and warm. The other patients didn't look as if they were struggling. They appeared to be doing fine. They were getting chemotherapy, that's all. They were doing fine. And so looking back, you know, I had a memory of such a pleasant experience. Of course, I see Yumi sitting there, Yigal is sitting there, your tapes are playing. And the view is gorgeous.

I traveled in my mind, to that first night, with all the vomiting. Of course, my first stop is Lake Barf, but it brings only laughter...I don't feel nauseous. Getting back into the car and driving until I vomit again, is still fine. I'm not feeling nauseous; what I'm feeling is love. I'm remembering Yigal in the car, saying, "All is well, Mom and Dad, I'm right here, all is well. I'm not afraid." And it was so clear he wasn't afraid. He was giving us that fearless love. He was so fully present and "there" for us both. There's more vomiting, followed by your soft, soothing voice filling the car with your wonderful guided imagery. We arrive at our destination, to find stuffed bears, food, letters, and hearts. It feels like an invitation to wholeness. Yumi says he feels carried on the wings of angels. I just start crying...feeling the same thing...carried on the wings of angels, people's prayers, their support, the energetic mail that I received internationally. I feel so uplifted. This is the first time I've ever needed this kind of support; it's all new to me. The whole place is packed with love, down to the last detail. Loving support is pouring in from everywhere. "Carried on the wings of angels"...Yumi's expression was so perfect. Because that's exactly the sensation. No vomiting or nausea in my mental journey.

*The positive e-mail updates that Louise kept sending created a massive flow of prayers and good wishes for your well-being.*

It was palpable. I have that as a positive touchstone as well. I think that the research they've done on people's immune system following chemotherapy, was done on people who did not have a support system in place, to this extent. They had a lot of fear energy. I think that fearless love energy is such a powerful, powerful thing. And I had a lot of that. Including my son's fearless love. Where did he get it?

And then there's another angel, my mom. The other day I called her. Just listening to how much she loves me, and she loves life, and she loves being alive, and she loves that my voice is in the telephone...the power of her spirit is awesome. Her memory is very, very bad now, but her spirit, and her positiveness is as powerful as it ever was. It's just incredible. I couldn't stop crying, just thinking about how wonderful I feel with her.

# Chapter 17

# Rituals

There have been so many rituals that have served to refocus me during my journey. They truly helped me to embrace the event more fully.

***The Letter Ritual...***When I got your letter I began dancing in the parking lot. Up to that point, Yumi and I were feeling our way along each day; we had made a decision that this is an event and that it needs to be embraced. We knew we were in charge of how it would unfold. We had begun assigning playful names of "rallying around the boob" and "the boob brigade" for all those who were showing up to help. We were really creating a whole language that I deeply resonated to. The term "cellular challenge" was so perfect. We knew this cellular challenge represented an adventure for both of us, and we intended to dance through it in a way that included a spirit of celebration at every possible moment. But, until your letter arrived, no one had put what we were doing into words. You expressed to perfection just what we were doing and how I was feeling. People were calling this cellular challenge the Big "C" and to me it felt like the little "c" with a BIG "ME." But, in feeling that way, I was also aware that I was all alone in my viewpoint. As I read your letter, I was so thrilled that I went out into the parking lot of our condominium and danced. *[laughter]* I just danced all around the parking lot out of pure joy.

Then I began taking your letter with me wherever we went. If I got distracted from our path, or the focus that we had, I would reread the letter, and it would get me right on the path again. You know, if we were in a waiting room, and I forgot that this is the place for me to have fun right now, I would read your letter, and find the fun in that moment. So your letter was just a wonderful refocus-er, you know. Rereading it provided a ritual that got me right back on track, over, and over, and over again. It was absolutely wonderful.

***The Ritual of the Magic Wand...***This was such a simple, profound, fresh, new perspective to embrace as I felt my way through this entire journey. Taking my "invisible magic wand" everywhere I went on this journey was so clarifying. It seemed to quickly cut through the confusion and place my attention solidly on what I wanted. Even when I kept flipping back to the drama, once I realized that I had gone there, I instantly knew where to head. My work in the moment was always the same... to feel my way to a better-feeling place. Just knowing that there always is a better-feeling place seemed to accelerate the process. I am never without my wand! It's an ongoing ritual. What a gift.

***The Ritual of Story-Telling...***The day that I was to receive "the news" from the doctor was the perfect day to tell my staff the story of the black belt that my client had presented to me. They were so frightened for me. Telling that story not only centered me, but centered my staff as well. I took my time and told every detail. It was the perfect touchstone to remember the healer inside of me. After that, I was ready to "slowly" get the news. I would take my time and be fully present for the trip to the doctor's office. I would be centered as I received "the news."

***The Ritual of the Circle of Women...***This turned out to have a totally different benefit than I originally thought it would have. Initially, I thought it would be a ceremony to usher me into the next step of my journey which was (chemo) therapy. It was a circle of dear friends—but friends who were seized with fear about what was ahead in my journey. It quickly became a circle of fear. <u>They</u> needed the circle to find their balance regarding my journey. And I needed them to take on a lighter style of support than most of them had ever known. You played a major role in initiating them into a way of thinking and speaking that was admittedly a stretch for them. But, it gave them a rhythm for the future that would help them support me in ways that I truly resonated to. They learned to speak a little more of the language of well-being and celebration...and gradually moved further from the language of solemn-ness and fear. They learned to giggle and laugh about life even when it was paired with a diagnosis of cancer. They learned to sing a new note that matched mine. It was a powerful and pivotal experience.

***The Ritual of Preparing the Condo...***Louise turned that beach condo into a magnificent message that said, "Welcome to Wholeness." "All Is Well!" Every detail had been thought of. Friends had prepared food so that we wouldn't have to cook. They provided a juicer for nourishing drinks. There were bears, hearts, and letters, and the place was just filled with loving support. And Yumi said he felt "carried on the wings of angels." I said, "That's exactly right." It was the perfect place to focus on wellness.

***The Ritual of Cutting Hair...***This was such an empowering event. I chose how I would embrace this portion of my experience. "<u>I</u> happened to it," rather than letting "<u>it</u> happen to me." I got the jump on it! I lost it purposefully, with loving support in all directions. My hairdresser and friend, Ruth, playfully unveiled a parade of different "me's" as she played with this style and that on the way to the final half inch, crew cut version. She cut it long on one side—short on the other, short in the back—long in the front, bangs to one side, full bangs, etc., as my hair gradually became shorter and shorter. Part of the ceremony included a blessing for my whole body, which was so important. It was critical that I remembered that this is only part of my life, my hair is part of something greater (my body); and my body is part of something even greater, my spirit. I am not my hair. It was extremely freeing, as if a looming concern had suddenly dissolved and was quickly replaced by radiance.

***The Ritual of the Sabbath...***There is nothing more delightful to us than the ritual of welcoming the Sabbath and stopping everything to just allow Spirit to renew us. We thoroughly enjoy all the preparation: the shopping for food, preparing the food, the flowers, the prayers, the meals—all of this adds to the sacredness of the day. It truly provides an ongoing fuel for us in all we do. Even when I was low in energy, Yumi would do all the preparation, and I still went downstairs to participate in as much as I could. It was fuel for my soul. In honoring the Sabbath, we were continually fueled with the sacred.

***The Ritual of Expanding Rituals...***You know, my son Avi, and daughter-in-law Sharon, provided a tremendous blessing for us during their visit. In Israel, they are totally devoted to their religious beliefs. The seminary has been an extraordinary experience for Avi. They absolutely love their life there, honor and love the rules (of which there are tons!) and they live a very sacred life. It's so beautiful to see them. But the rules also make traveling quite complicated and stressful when they go outside of the seminary. The Kosher Choreographer inspired them to notice a book that was full of tips on how to become flexible with your family members who are not of the same religious orientation. This expansion of their rituals meant that they came with a new willingness to be flexible. They were absolutely wonderful about blending into our household. They were so generous, and loved us so much, that they expanded their religious rituals into a less structured form for the entire visit. What a blessing!

***The Ritual of Greeting Cards...***"Toss and keep, toss and keep." You know, I truly had to keep only the cards and notes that I resonated to. Only the ones that empowered me. But that collection of cards became a delight to look through, again and again. Notes referring to my "inner strength," or my "creative ability to find the good in all situations," or that "angels were traveling everywhere with me, smoothing my journey." Even though I quickly tossed the ones that I did not resonate to, I was careful to extract the good intentions that were sent with them. People mean well, they just don't always know appropriate and helpful things to say. I would translate their notes into things like, "They want me to know they love and support me in this journey." Then I'd toss the card, and keep the thoughtfulness!

***The Ritual of Celebration...***Well, as you know, this was the common theme on my entire journey. Celebration was and is my way of truly "living" in the moment. Why wait? There are things to celebrate now. Depending on what was possible at the time, I celebrated by choosing favorite foods, wearing special outfits, buying something special (even a new mattress!), shopping for clothes, seeing dear friends, writing wonderful notes of appreciation, relaxing at a beach condo, listening to the ocean, listening to my favorite music, dining in a favorite restaurant, and visiting Yumi's father. After each doctor's appointment, after every single radiation treatment, we would find a way to celebrate. When I was finishing the last few days of radiation, it was common to hear friends say, "You must have a celebration after that last treatment!" I said, "Oh, I'm not waiting to celebrate then. I've celebrated every single day of treatment." It had never occurred to them to celebrate "on the way" to where you are going. They only knew of celebrating the arrival at the end of the journey. This ritual of celebrating "now" is just very connecting.

***The Ritual of Translation...***I not only translated negative greetings in cards into the true message behind the gesture, but I translated conversations everywhere I went. The ritual of transforming the words that are spoken by well-meaning people, and turning them into what they really mean so that they serve in the way they were intended, is truly a transformational process. People would refer to my "sickness" and I didn't feel sick; or they would refer to "my cancer" instead of my "diagnosis of cancer" in which I didn't establish ownership. It's not about denial; it's just not the language I resonate to. While it's really nice not to have the reference to "sickness," "disease," "your cancer," or "overwhelming times," I found that I could instantly change it by silently restating what I knew they really meant. What she really means is, "I love Hedy and I'm really thinking about her, and I'm sending her marvelous energy and thinking of her as vibrantly alive and well." I practice the ritual of translation wherever I go. I've become a "translation specialist!"

***The Ritual of Appreciation...***You know, there has been an unending stream of things I've appreciated in this journey. What I want to say here, is how much I've appreciated the unending support you have given to Yumi and me during our journey. You put your marvelous words to what we were already doing intuitively. You continually held a space for me at the star end of the wand. Any time I went for a slide (to the stick end), you greeted me as I returned to the star. You sang a steady note that I thoroughly resonated to. You joined me in celebration. You joined me in finding what I would say "Yes!" to in life. You provided such incredibly simple ways to behold life, even in it's most complicated moments. You were always about empowering, clarifying, simplifying and rejoicing. You gave splendid new meaning to "magic wands," "valves" and "cookies!" I will never be the same, my friend. For this, and so much more, I will continue the ritual of appreciation, as Yumi and I travel about in our work. It is with enormous love, appreciation and admiration, that I say, in outrageous aliveness, goodbye for now!

# Chapter 18

# Caughtcha!
## A New Beginning at The End

*All right, I confess...I have the habit of flipping to the last chapter of new books and peeking at that first. (Books on algebra and calculus are exceptions.) If you've just now flipped to this last chapter, Hello! (Caughtcha!) If not, then hopefully by now you're sporting a distinct glow from having read* Sacred Choices—*a glow that reflects the sensation of having received the profound "massage" that was offered as a gift just for you:*

*a massage of your perceptions in life,*
  *a massage of your reality,*
    *and most importantly,*
      *a massage of your empowerment and Authenticity!*

*My priceless friend, Kay Visser, puts it like this:*

*"*Sacred Choices *is a 'feel-good story' about 'feel-bad subjects'!"*

*You know, my greatest wish for you is that you remember who you really are. Remember? You are a Spiritual being having a silly/ profound, temporary human experience...just for the fun of it. (God loves the silly—lighten up!) Each of us is equipped with a state-of-the art, built-in guidance system. It was specially designed by our Creator to guide us through every situation in the best possible way, whether we're wondering which restaurant to go to, or what action to take following a frightening diagnosis. This finely-tuned system employs our emotions as an "invisible meter," which continually tells us where we reside in this ongoing game of spiritual connection. Joy is the infallible sign of the presence of God. When you are feeling emotions of Joy, appreciation, love, etc., it's a sure sign that you're well-connected and your meter is pointing to "fully alive!" Now imagine what the feelings of resentment, blame, regret, worry, and fear indicate on your meter. Since God won't join you in blaming and hating, etc., it's the "little you" trying very hard to make life work. You wonder why you feel emotionally drained and physically tired. Your meter is pointing to "life-less" or should I say "less life."*

*Being spiritually aligned does not mean that you side-step all challenging moments. It means that you have the ability to deal with everything from a higher perspective—by feeling your way along with your guidance system. I love the fact that when you're "connected" it automatically sprinkles your day with those synchronistic moments in which you "accidentally" stumble across precisely what you need. I'm sure it's a form of entertainment for angels. The very same afternoon that I realized my mother would be needing an assisted living facility, I found that the administrator of the perfect facility was standing next to me at a furniture store. I had never met her before but was inspired to say "Hello" while we were waiting in line together at the cashier. It was a spontaneous, celestially-orchestrated chat, timed to perfection by unseen helpers. (The same ones that I suspect were getting a good laugh out of watching the event unfold.) The other synchronistic thing was that they just happened to have a bed available in a room that was perfect for my mother...and I found it all at the furniture store. (Perhaps the sign on the front of the store should read..."Furniture—And Much, Much More!") How I love those synchronistic moments! I've found that the more that I notice them, and the more I expect them, the more they occur. It's also nice to remember to say, "Thank you!" to these unseen helpers. It's a relationship worth nourishing.*

*Can you maintain your balance even while tragic events are surfacing like the Oklahoma bombing, ethnic cleansing in Kosovo, and the shooting rampage at Columbine High School? Is it possible to watch the evening news and feel good all the way through? You tell me...the answer is in* Sacred Choices.

*As far as your health is concerned, along with whatever treatment you are inspired to choose, one Rx remains a powerful complement in every case:*

*Rx:* • *Be sensitive to how you are feeling in each moment.*

• *Continually look for thoughts that feel better.*

• *Remember that nothing is more important than that you feel good emotionally.*

• *Never miss a chance to laugh and appreciate.*

• *Speak to yourself like a loving, supportive good friend. Your cells are listening!*

*Over the years, research has shown this "body/mind connection" to be undeniable. What you mentally anticipate stimulates a wave of changes in the body on a cellular level. Think for a moment of chomping into a large wedge of a lemon. Come on now, take a nice big bite out of that wedge. Notice the juice from that tart, lemony pulp exploding in your mouth each time your teeth bite down on it. Unless you are taking medications that dry your mouth, just the thought of chewing the lemon normally triggers an immediate flood of saliva! Isn't that fascinating? The software that came with the cells in our bodies is awesome.*

*In the same way that our cells are programmed to respond to our thoughts and emotions, they're also programmed to automatically seek balance and health. You might say that if you were able to get your "judgmental self" or your "negative self" out of the way, your cells would just naturally move towards wellness. But first, you must become aware of whatever opinions and thoughts are holding you back; things you are resenting, fearing, worrying about, etc. Your job is to get out of the way. You get out of the way* *when you choose thoughts that feel good. You get out of the way when you label any negative emotion for what it is (fear, anger, resentment), stop resisting it, and let it pass on through. (Chapter 16) You get out of the way when you speak a language that supports wholeness. (Chapter 1) You get out of the way by choosing physicians, healthcare settings and healthcare staff (the entire package) <u>that you resonate with</u>, instead of "fearfully or dutifully showing-up" for an appointment assigned by your referring physician. (Chapter 4) You get out of the way when you choose a plan for your well-being and health that feels just right for you. You get out of the way when you find creative ways to align yourself with upcoming tests or treatments prior to your arrival. Your inner alignment in every case is the critical ingredient.*

*Contrary to popular belief, there are no celestial points for just tolerating or enduring life. This is not an endurance test. This is not a test, period! Has it ever occurred to you that all this stuff you call "life" could be about nothing more than "finding the fun"? That's another way of saying, "finding God in all things." It's about being fully alive and fully present. Many don't start to live until they're face-to-face with their own mortality. (Now we can really make some choices—sacred choices!)*

*Is it possible to feel physically uncomfortable and yet feel spiritually outstanding at the same time? You tell me...the answer is written in* Sacred Choices. *Is it possible to prepare yourself ahead of time so that you maintain your spiritual connection during doctor's visits, CAT scans, MRI's, biopsies, surgery, chemotherapy, radiation, lab tests, etc., and emerge feeling whole and balanced? Absolutely. However, nothing is more important than having the Connected You show up in every case. Even simpler...nothing is more important than that you find thoughts that feel good, moment to moment. Just out of curiosity...how ARE you feeling in this moment? Have you found any fun yet?*

*Admittedly, something that's synonymous with healthcare is "waiting." Waiting is that often pesky / miserable / stifling / downtime that most people think they must endure.*

*People are:*

  *waiting to graduate,*

    *waiting to get married,*

      *waiting to get divorced,*

        *waiting for the perfect job,*

          *waiting to get well,*

            *waiting to complete chemotherapy,*

              *waiting for the last dose of radiation,*

              *waiting for the perfect mate,*

              *waiting to get pregnant,*

              *waiting to get thinner,*

                *waiting on the telephone to speak*
                *to their insurance company,*

                *waiting for the check to arrive,*

              *waiting for the lab results, and*

            *waiting for the waiting to be over.*

*We fool ourselves into thinking that the most important part lies at the end of the wait. While the goal may be quite significant, it's not necessarily the most important part. The "wait" itself potentially contains a profound gift. It could actually be considered the main event. You've probably heard the expression that "joy is in the journey." We tend to think of any journey as "going some place" and that perhaps it takes a long time; but I want to suggest that if you're stricken with panic for two minutes while sitting right in your living room, you've been on quite a journey. There are journeys, and there are journeys!*

*Waiting is a journey; you're traveling from where you find yourself emotionally to whatever you have your sight set on, at the end of the wait. It's the waiting game. But, rather than play the game, many choose to merely endure the whole process, and in doing so they miss the main event. The joy is in the wait! The fun is in the wait. God is in the wait.*

*The rules in the waiting game are simple. First, you must realize that the game has begun! It's so easy to get consumed with the drama and totally miss the starting bell. Then you simply find ways to maintain a "feel-good" state during the wait, and you win—big time! Actually, you even get points for brief periods of "feeling good" during the wait, just as long as you keep pursuing your connection. Whether it's a two-minute wait while on hold on the telephone or a 48-hour wait for lab results, we weren't meant to disconnect from home base, tapping our foot impatiently until God shows up with the goods!*

*A friend of mine got the shock of her life when she returned home to find that her 15-year-old son had stolen the family car and run away from home with a buddy of his. Her son is a bit developmentally slow and had failed his driving test three times. She was admittedly hoping he'd never pass because she worried that he just wasn't quick enough to drive safely. Now she was filled with worries from every angle. He might get into an accident, someone might harm him or try to take advantage of him, he might harm someone else in an accident, he might get hurt, he might get arrested for driving without a license. Who knew what could happen? The list was endless and she was overwhelmed with fright.*

*Earlier that same day, she had attended my workshop on "Joy 101." She soon remembered a technique that I teach called "rocking." It's a powerful tool that's perfect for waiting and for those helpless moments. Since we're all connected and love knows no boundaries, this technique is ideal for reaching someone from a distance. The first step is to drop all other agendas and admit that you truly want to be of help. (In my friend's case, it's not the time to be thinking of what consequences to give him when he returns home!) Then you picture this person as they would look at three months old. You merely put this innocent little three-month-old over your shoulder and rock him for a little over a minute with the message that "all is well." (Chapter 5)*

*"All is well?" you say! How can all be well if he's out risking life and limb (and car)? Well, what that means is that you are*

*supporting and energetically joining the very best in him. In other words, you are focusing on and embracing his spiritually connected self. While he's on his adventure, you have a choice. You can either energetically hang on his ankles in fear (fear also knows no boundaries) or choose to be the wind beneath his wings. In choosing "all is well," you are saying that you embrace the part of him that thinks clearly and makes good decisions. You want him to feel your love; you want him to be steady and wise beyond his years. If he's chosen to experience an adventure, you want him to make good choices. All of that is summed up in the statement "all is well." It's simple, profound, connecting, and the perfect thing for a helpless moment in which you must wait. You rock this three-month-old infant back and forth, reminding him of his magnificence and remembering yours as well. The most important ingredient is the steady, pure focus. You only need to do it for a little over a minute. She rocked him all night long.*

*By embracing someone on this level, you've simultaneously found your own spiritual connection; so there's a second benefit in that you also slide to the star end of life's magic wand during the wait. I spoke to her on the following day and learned that not only was she doing well, but she had never seen such a calm response in her husband during a crisis. She said normally, he would have been her second problem! He would have been angry, frustrated and out of control. But keep in mind that he was sleeping in bed right beside her as she mentally rocked her son and silently chanted "all is well" throughout the night. No wonder he was calm! It gave her even more confidence that this technique was truly making a difference. Her husband said, "I figure when he gets tired enough, hungry enough, and runs out of money, he'll be back." She thought, "Who IS this man?!" Her son returned home safely on the third day. They each had a phenomenal journey. God was in each journey. God was in the wait! She chose to be the wind beneath her son's wings. (Then she grounded him! That's a mother for you.)*

*Techniques for sustaining your connection vary for every occasion and every person:*

Listen to your favorite uplifting music,
see a funny movie,
call a good friend,
take a walk,
go for a run,
go for a drive,
breathe deeply and sigh long sighs,
take a hot bath...light candles around the tub,
sing,
play with a child,
dance (even if you can only dance in your mind),
have a massage,
meditate,
paint,
celebrate the moment,
celebrate anything,
shop,
pet a puppy or kitten,
journal your fondest memories,
write lists of things you appreciate,
rock a three-month-old version of yourself,
wink and wave to yourself in the mirror
(even better if it's a mirror adjacent
to the department store escalator),
swing on a swing,
blow bubbles,
lie in the grass and watch clouds,
eat something fabulous,
talk to yourself about it until it feels better,
or (for those who've read the chapter on "The
Dance of Remembrance") shout "Cookies! This
is just more cookies!" "Let's see...what do I
want more of?" (Write it down.)

*No matter what the diagnosis is or what the lab tests show, to be flooded with Life Force in any moment means that there has been a cellular shift towards health and well-being. Now that's empowerment. That's the way to wait! God's waiting patiently for you to get the hang of this kind of waiting. It's a choice. He also gives you free will to choose disconnection. Whatever! It's your breath.*

*My friend Kay shared these personally-empowering highlights from* Sacred Choices:

- Doubt and fear were meant to serve as 'cues'—
  not as lifestyles.

- Perception is the only thing we can truly control.

- The perfect question is, "What's another way I can
  look at this?"

- I get more of whatever I give my attention to.

- There is light…and the absence of light…but there
  is no darkness.

- As I open up more to life, it opens up to me.

- I can <u>choose</u> to reference the good times and the good stuff.

- "Fearless" love is a powerful healer.

- I can send e-mail (energetic mail) without a computer!
  I can bathe people in peace and well-being by holding that
  vision in my thoughts. We are all invisibly connected.

- I don't have to try to stop thinking negatively…I merely need
  to turn my attention to what I am wanting and visually
  embrace all aspects of it. Since I can't hold negative thoughts
  and positive thoughts simultaneously,  there is automatically
  no room for the negative thought.

- Rather than claim a disease as mine ("my arthritis," "my
  cancer," "I have cancer."), it's beneficial to say that "I was
  diagnosed with arthritis," etc., recognize it as "just passing
  through!"

- Being positive is not about painting black—white. It is not about trying to suppress the negative. It's about giving my attention to what connects me on an emotional level with who I really am and letting go of resistance.

- I can easily spot areas of negativity and resistance merely by being sensitive to how I'm feeling in the moment. My emotions serve as my built-in guidance system for finding and maintaining my spiritual connection.

- My body naturally seeks balance and well-being. The best thing I can do is get out of the way by letting go of resistance and thoughts that aren't serving me well.

- The Language of Well-being is the language of health and wholeness. My cells are listening and responding. I loved the example of substituting the term "cellular challenge" for the word "cancer!" "Cellular challenge" clearly feels better.

- In terms of grieving the loss of a loved one, the pain ceases the minute my full attention is on wonderful moments we shared together. When I'm fully re-living and re-loving one of those moments (as opposed to noticing that those moments are now gone), it is impossible to simultaneously feel the loss. It's a powerful choice.

- My body is continually responding to my emotions.

- Before setting foot out of bed in the morning, I want to affirm that, "Nothing is more important than that I feel good." AND that, "No matter what happens today, I'm going to find ways to keep my valve (to my well-being) wide open."

*Finding our spiritual connection during moments of major disconnection means regaining that sense of aliveness and empowerment. It means thriving instead of surviving. It means soaring spiritually even while your child is missing. In the case of a life-threatening diagnosis, it means choosing life and aliveness instead of being consumed with "trying not to die." It means exercising because "you're worth it" and you love taking good care of yourself (star end of the wand), instead of trying to fend off death (stick end of the wand). Your body knows the difference. Or, in the case of a terminal illness, it means being fully alive right up to the moment of rebirth and radical aliveness on the other side. Slipping into your Authentic Self (the spiritually connected "You") means that you live with an awareness that there is something greater happening—a bigger picture, and that you look for the potential blessing (the punch line) contained in everything. It means embracing each journey—whether it's two minutes, two years or two decades.*

*So—there you have it...life being lived by the simple truth that, "Nothing is more important than that I feel good." In living that truth, no matter what challenge is going on in my life, I always know how to find clarity, flow, and inspiration, and I'm unrelenting in my pursuit. Finding creative and fun ways to spiritually connect in each moment remains my passion. For me it represents the "simple that's absolutely oozing with the profound." Yes, at the end of this lifetime tour I want to be able to say that "I did it"—I remembered to seek my spiritual connection right in the middle of regular daily life...whether it was while bagging potatoes in the produce department of the grocery store or holding my mother's hand as she lay dying. I want to be able to say that I embraced my spiritual connection not only in the ordinary moments of life, but even in the midst of extraordinary, potentially disconnecting moments. I continue to adore the epitaph that I've chosen for myself which says it all. It reads:*

*"I Remembered!"*

The Beginning.

## *And They Lived Happily Ever After!*

*Hedy and Yumi are traveling internationally while teaching the Imago Workshops originated by Harville Hendrix...author of* Getting The Love You Want. *She is a "Fearless Mama"...laughing and celebrating all that life brings, and is truly the Pied Piper of Joy. Her workshops and clinical training have a "New Hedy" that is more empowered than ever, and consequently, the work being done by the participants is even more profound. She and Yumi continue to celebrate life and are living happily ever after!*

*Whenever possible, you'll still find Judie sporting her favorite t-shirt, shorts, and Reeboks (no accessories)...teaching, writing, laughing, massaging (bodies and perceptions), doing "trashercise" on daily walks, attending Carl's softball games, playing often in the bushes and flowers, invisibly "rocking" this one and that one (anyone with a pulse!), using television news broadcasts to practice "valvular aerobics," looking for things to appreciate, occasionally checking out the "stick end of the wand" for brief periods, choosing her favorite "cookies" each day, and living with a passionate goal of "remembering to remember" who she is, even in the most casual and ordinary of circumstances. Years ago she was diagnosed as having a full-blown and highly contagious case of "radical aliveness!"*

# *Notes*

### Chapter 1: The Dance of Remembrance

1. (page 39)  For more on the mind/body connection see pages 27-31 in *Women's Bodies, Women's Wisdom* by Christiane Northrup; also pages 31-32 *Return to Wholeness* by David Simon.

2. (page 41)  For more on the mind/body connection see pages 27-31 in *Women's Bodies, Women's Wisdom* by Christiane Northrup; also pages 31-32 in *Return to Wholeness* by David Simon.

3. (page 45)  Maurice Chevalier sang, "I Remember, Yes I Remember," in the 1950's Broadway musical *Gigi*.

4. (page 49)  The *Jewish Talmud* is a book composed of the early authoritative religious writings that form the basis of orthodox Judaism.

### Chapter 2: Cookies!

1. (page 64)  Braille is a system of printing for the blind in which letters and numerals are represented by raised dots.

### Chapter 3: Rallying 'Round The Boob!

1. (page 73)  Woody Allen is an actor, comedian, director, musician and screenwriter.

### Chapter 4:  The Search For "The Boob Dream Team!"

1. (page 100)  Bolen, Jean Shinoda. *Close to the Bone, Life-Threatening Illness and the Search for Meaning.* New York, New York: Scribner, 1996.

2. (page 100)  The sentinel node is a lymph node that is said to be the "node on watch." This is the first lymph node to receive cancer cells. If it tests positive for cancer, there may be other positive nodes upstream. If this node is negative, all the upstream nodes are negative 99 out of 100 times.

### Chapter 5: Soul Food

1. (page 111)  *My Radiation Therapy Coloring Book—A Child's Eye View of Radiation Therapy* by Joi Cangelosi, Tina Miceli, Barbara Siede, Barbara Fineberg, The Ochsner Medical Foundation, New Orleans, 1516 Jefferson Highway, New Orleans, Louisiana 70121.

2. (page 113)  A Bone Scan is an x-ray done of the skeletal system using a radioactive dye. It is used to detect abnormalities in the bony structures of the body.

3. (page 113)  A CAT Scan (Computed Tomography Imaging Scan) is a method of making x-ray images of the interior of the body.

## Chapter 12:  Freedom to Soar

1. (page 228)  This teaching is from Abraham who teaches through Esther Hicks. I've consistently found the Abraham teachings to be very practical and effective for maintaining spiritual flow in daily life. For more information, write Abraham Hicks Publications, P.O. Box 690070, San Antonio, TX 78269.

2. (page 231)  Chakra is a Hindu word meaning "wheel of light." We have a number of chakras (also called energy centers) throughout our bodies. Generally, the focus is on seven major centers in the human torso, neck and head. Chakras have a natural spinning action that generate an electromagnetic (or auric field) around the body. A wonderful reference for further studies on chakras is *Wheels of Light* by Rosalyn Bruyere.

## Chapter 14:  The Incessant Demand For Radical Aliveness

1. (page 257)  Author and medical intuitive, Carolyn Myss, coined the term "woundology."

2. (page 260)  Moss, Richard. *The Black Butterfly, an Invitation to Radical Aliveness.* Berkeley, California: Celestial Arts, 1986. (page 60)

3. (page 261)  Moss, Richard. *The Black Butterfly, an Invitation to Radical Aliveness.* Berkeley, California: Celestial Arts, 1986. (page 60)

4. (page 261)  Moss, Richard. *The Black Butterfly, an Invitation to Radical Aliveness.* Berkeley, California: Celestial Arts, 1986. (page 64)

5. (page 262)  Tai Chi is the ancient Chinese martial arts system of exercise. It has the quality of a dance that's performed in slow motion. Tai Chi is known for stimulating energy flow as it takes the body through a full range of motion.

6. (page 264) Steven Spielberg founded the Shoah Visual History Foundation in 1994. It was formed to record the amazing stories of survival during the holocaust, and to preserve them for history.

## Chapter 15: Perception is a Choice

1. (page 277)  A Moxibustion stick is a wand made of slow-burning herbs. It's often used to enhance the effects of acupuncture. The hot tip is used to warm the acupuncture needle, further stimulating the area being treated.

2. (page 277)  Chakra is a Hindu word meaning "wheel of light." We have a number of chakras (also called energy centers) throughout our bodies. Generally, the focus is on seven major centers in the human torso, neck and head. Chakras have a natural spinning action that generate an electromagnetic or (auric field) around the body. A wonderful reference for further studies on chakras is *Wheels of Light* by Rosalyn Bruyere.

## Chapter 16:  Soul Illumination

1. (308) Iyanla Vanzant writes about "crying with an agenda" in her book, *Yesterday I Cried...Celebrating the Lessons of Living and Loving.* 1999

# Suggested Reading

Bolen, Jean Shinoda. *Close to the Bone, Life-Threatening Illness and the Search for Meaning*. New York, New York: Scribner, 1996.

Chiappone, Judie. *The Light Touch...an Easy Guide to Hands-on-Healing*. Winter Springs, Florida: Holistic Reflections, Inc., 1989.

Ban Breathnach, Sarah. *Simple Abundance*. New York, New York: Warner Books, Inc., 1995.

Carlson, Richard. *Don't Sweat The Small Stuff...And It's All Small Stuff*. New York, New York: Hyperion Press, 1997.

Chopra, Deepak. *Ageless Body, Timeless Mind*. New York, New York: Crown Publishers, Inc., 1993.

Gray, John. *How to Get What You Want and Want What You Have: A Practical and Spiritual Guide to Personal Success*, New York, New York: Harper Collins, 1999.

Hicks, Esther and Jerry. *Sara and The Foreverness of Friends of a Feather*. San Antonio, Texas: Abraham-Hicks Publications, 1995.

Hicks, Esther and Jerry. *Sara and Seth, Solomon's Fine Featherless Friends*. San Antonio, Texas: Abraham-Hicks Publications, 1999.

Moss, Richard. *The Black Butterfly, an Invitation to Radical Aliveness*. Berkeley, California: Celestial Arts, 1986.

Northrup, Christiane. *Women's Bodies, Women's Wisdom*. New York, New York: Bantam, 1998.

O'Donnell, Rosie, and Deborah Axelrod. *Bosom Buddies...Lessons and Laughter on Breast Health and Cancer*. New York, New York: Time Warner, 1999.

Remen, Rachel Naomi. *Kitchen Table Wisdom, Stories That Heal*. New York, New York: Riverhead Books, 1996.

Sark. *Inspirational Sandwich*. Berkeley, California: Celestial Arts, 1988.

Simon, David. *Return to Wholeness...Embracing Body, Mind, and Spirit in the Face of Cancer*. New York, New York: John Wiley and Sons, Inc., 1999.

Vanzant, Iyanla. *One Day My Soul Just Opened Up*. New York, New York: Fireside, 1998.

Weil, Andrew. *Spontaneous Healing: How to Discover and Enhance Your Body's Natural Ability to Maintain and Heal Itself*. New York, New York: Knopf, 1995.

# About the Author

Judie Chiappone is a gifted teacher, noted for her ability to inspire others into greater wholeness and healing. She is a dynamic and entertaining speaker, passionate about showing others how to sustain their spiritual connection in everyday living. As a Registered Nurse and Licensed Massage Therapist, Judie has physically and spiritually touched and enhanced the lives of thousands. She is the author of *The Light Touch..an Easy Guide to Hands-on-Healing,* as well as an empowering, guided-imagery tape entitled, *Sacred Choices for Chemotherapy.* Judie lives with her husband Carl in Winter Springs, Florida.

## How to contact the author...

Holistic Reflections, Inc.
Judie Chiappone
P.O. Box 196129
Winter Springs, FL 32719-6129

Phone: (407) 327-7777

web site: www.SacredChoices.com
e-mail: Judie@SacredChoices.com

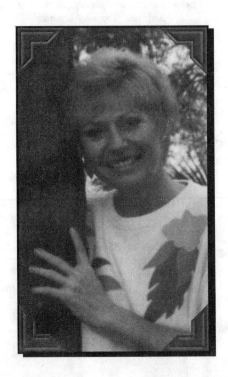